TABLE OF CONTENTS

INTRODUCTION

PURPOSE OF THE BOOK

In today's busy world, trying to be healthy and happy can feel like a fight against time and false information. There are so many quick fixes and fad diets out there that many people feel confused and let down. This book, which is mostly about chair yoga for weight loss, wants to bring back the idea of overall well-being, which means that the goal is not just to lose weight but also to keep the mind, body, and spirit in balance.

Why do chair yoga?

Chair yoga stands out as an easy-to-use and useful tool on this path to better health. There are many good things about traditional yoga, but it can be scary or hard for people who are just starting out, have physical limits, or are overweight. Chair yoga is a kinder, more inclusive option that lets more people experience the deep benefits of yoga. The goal of this book is to take the mystery out of yoga and make it easy for everyone to do, no matter their fitness level, age, or body type.

Trying to lose weight by being mindful and moving

The point of this book is to show people how to do a set of chair yoga poses that are especially made to help them lose weight. The method is not just physical, though. While chair yoga is a gentle but effective way to work out, it also presents the idea of emotional and mental health as important parts of losing weight. This book describes methods that are meant to make you more aware of your body, help you deal with stress (which can make you gain weight), and help you form healthier habits.

Educational and Enabling

The goal of this book is to teach people not only the poses and routines of chair yoga, but also the ideas behind yoga that can be used in everyday life. Readers can take charge of their health journey if they understand the "why" behind each movement and breathing method. This book aims to bring about a change on the inside and the outside by giving information and tools.

A Complete Guide for Long-Term Weight Loss

This book takes a broad view of weight loss because it knows that it's a process that involves more than just exercise. It will talk about eating, making changes to your lifestyle, and mental health. These are all very important for losing weight and staying at a healthy weight. In order to help people lose weight in a healthy way that will last, the book stays away from extreme diets and intense exercise plans, which don't always work in the long run.

Adaptable and unique

One of the best things about this book is that it can be changed to fit different needs. Because everyone's body and weight loss process is different, the book shows how to change different yoga poses and sequences to fit each person's strengths and weaknesses. This personalized method makes sure that anyone who reads this book can use chair yoga to help them lose weight.

Final Thoughts

In the end, this book's goal is to give you a complete, easy-to-use, and long-lasting way to lose weight through chair yoga. Its goal is to teach, inspire, and assist people on their path to better health, stressing the significance of a balanced approach that cares for the mind, body, and spirit all at the same time. People who finish this book should not only know how to do yoga, but also have a new outlook on health and wellness that can change their lives.

BENEFITS OF CHAIR YOGA FOR WEIGHT LOSS

Chair yoga is a gentle form of yoga that can be done sitting down on a chair or standing up with the help of a chair. It has a lot of health benefits, especially for people who want to lose weight and get healthier generally. This part goes into detail about the many ways that chair yoga can help you lose weight and improve your physical and mental health.

Adaptability and accessibility

One great thing about chair yoga is that it's easy to do. Traditional yoga poses can be hard to do, especially for people who are new to exercise, have trouble moving around, or are overweight. Chair yoga is a friendly option that makes yoga's benefits available to everyone. Everyone can do it and get the benefits because it can be changed to fit different body types and exercise levels.

Better metabolic function

Chair yoga can help you lose weight by changing the way your body works. Gentle exercises and stretches can help your digestive system work better and speed up your metabolism, both of which are important for losing weight. The exercise makes the body burn calories more efficiently, which helps with slow, long-term weight loss.

More toned and strong muscles

Even though it is easy, chair yoga is a good way to tone and strengthen your muscles. Even if the poses and moves are small, they still require muscles to be used. Over time, this makes muscles stronger and more toned, which helps burn fat and changes the way the body looks generally.

More flexibility and better joint health

Chair yoga improves flexibility and joint health when done regularly. This is especially helpful for people who are overweight, since being overweight can put stress on the joints and make them stiff and hurt. Better joint health and flexibility make it easier to move around, which makes other types of exercise easier to do and more fun.

Improving Heart and Blood vessel health

Because it involves flow and movement, chair yoga can be good for your heart. A key part of losing weight and improving your general health is having a healthier heart. Some chair yoga routines are meant to get your heart rate up, which gives your heart and lungs a light workout.

Less stress and better emotional health

A lot of people who are stressed out gain weight and eat poorly. Mindful breathing and relaxation techniques are used in chair yoga, and they help reduce worry and anxiety. A calmer mind helps you make better food choices and stops you from eating when you're stressed.

Better breathing efficiency

Chair yoga often focuses on breathing exercises that make the lungs work better. Better breathing increases the body's circulation, which helps the metabolism work faster and gives you more energy. As it helps the body work at its best, this can be especially helpful for losing weight.

More Mindfulness and Body Awareness

Chair yoga makes you more mindful and aware of your body. People who are more aware are better able to tell the difference between hunger and fullness, which keeps them from eating too much. Mindfulness also helps people eat better and develop healthy habits, which is a big help when trying to lose weight.

Less chance of getting chronic diseases

Chronic diseases like type 2 diabetes, high blood pressure, and heart disease are more likely to happen in people who are overweight or obese. Chair yoga can help lower the chance of these diseases. Chair yoga is a good way to manage and prevent these conditions because it gets you moving, lowers your stress, and improves your general health.

Chair yoga is a great way to get more energy and stamina in general. People with more energy may be more likely to be busy during the day, which helps them burn more calories, which is important for losing weight.

Building a Community That Helps Each Other

Chair yoga, especially when done with other people, can help people feel connected and supported. People who are trying to lose weight can benefit a lot from this support network, which can offer motivation, help, and the chance to share experiences.

To sum up, chair yoga has many benefits for people who want to lose weight and improve their health. It's easy for people of all ages, sizes, and exercise levels to do, and it can be changed to fit their needs. Chair yoga helps you lose weight in a healthy, long-term way by improving your metabolism, muscle tone, flexibility, circulatory and respiratory health, and lowering your stress. Mindfulness and body awareness are also improved through the exercise, which leads to healthier lifestyle choices and better overall health.

GETTING STARTED WITH CHAIR YOGA

MAKING YOUR ROOM READY FOR CHAIR YOGA

To start doing chair yoga, you need more than just a chair and a desire to learn. You also need a place that makes you feel calm, focused, and safe. This section is all about helping you make your chair yoga practice more enjoyable and successful. This is especially important for people who are using yoga to lose weight and improve their health.

Choosing the Right Place

Finding the right place is the first thing you need to do to get your space ready. This should ideally be a place that is quiet, clear, and doesn't get too much in the way. Just enough room to move your arms and legs around the chair without getting too squished. This could be a quiet spot in your bedroom, living room, or anywhere else.

Ensuring Enough Space

Make sure the area you pick is big enough to fit your chair and still let you move around easily. You shouldn't be able to bump into walls or furniture when you stretch your arms and legs out. For safety and ease of moving, there must be space around the chair.

Lighting and Sounds

Natural light is great for a yoga studio because it makes the place feel warm and inviting. If you can't get natural light, choose soft, relaxing artificial light. It's best to stay away from bright fluorescent lights because they can be annoying and unsettling. Soft-colored walls, candles, and plants can all improve the mood of your area and help you relax and concentrate.

Choosing a Chair That's Comfortable

In chair yoga, the chair is the most important piece of gear. Pick a strong chair that doesn't have arms so you can move around freely. The chair should have a flat seat and a back that supports you. Make sure it's the right height so that your knees are straight and your feet are flat on the floor.

Setting up a safe place to practice

Safety is very important. Make sure your chair doesn't move around during practice by putting it on a surface that won't slip. Put a yoga mat or a rug that won't slip under your chair if you're sitting on a smooth surface. Make sure there aren't any sharp or dangerous things close that you might hit by accident.

Making Your Space Your Own

Make your area your own to make it feel warm and welcoming and to help you relax and concentrate. Adding things that are important to you or make you feel calm, like photos, art, or symbols, could be part of this. But make sure that these personal touches don't make the room too crowded or take away from your practice.

Air flow and temperature

For a good yoga experience, the room should be at a comfortable temperature and have good air flow. It shouldn't be too hot or too cold in the room. If you can, practice in a room with windows that you can open to let in fresh air. But stay away from drafts that might bother you or take your attention away.

Audio and silence

If you find that quietness is relaxing, try to practice in a room that is away from noise from other rooms or at a time when it is quiet. On the other hand, nature sounds or soft background music can help you focus and relax during your practice. You could play soothing music on a small speaker or your phone.

Keeping yoga gear safe

Keep yoga gear like straps, blocks, and mats where they're easy to get to. Keeping your area clean and organized helps keep the peace and makes it easy to move from one pose or practice to the next.

Getting in the Mood

You might want to set the mood for each lesson before you start. For example, you could clean up for a few minutes, light a candle, play soft music, or take a few deep, relaxing breathes. Your body and mind may know that it's time to focus on your yoga practice when you do this routine.

Final Thoughts

Getting your room ready for chair yoga is an important first step. A well-kept area not only keeps you safe and comfortable, but it also makes your practice better overall. By making your space quiet, private, and free of distractions, you can have a meaningful and effective chair yoga lesson that is good for your physical and mental health and will help you reach your weight loss goals.

SAFETY TIPS AND MODIFICATIONS IN CHAIR YOGA

Chair yoga is usually a safe and easy way to work out, but you should still pay attention to safety to make sure you get the most out of the practice and don't hurt yourself. This part gives detailed safety instructions and suggestions for changes that can be made to fit people with different levels of ability and movement. This is especially important for people who are using chair yoga to lose weight and improve their health as a whole.

Understanding What Your Body Can't Do

To do chair yoga safely, you should first know and accept what your body can and can't do. It's important to know how fit you are, how flexible you are, and if you have any health problems or accidents. Before starting a new exercise plan, you should always talk to your doctor, especially if you have any long-term health problems or worries.

How to Pick the Right Chair

For safe chair yoga, it's important to choose the right chair. Pick a strong chair that doesn't have wheels. Arms shouldn't be on the chair because they can make it hard to move. The chair should be at a height where your feet are flat on the ground and your knees are bent about 90 degrees. Put a cushion or block under your feet if they don't reach the floor.

Heat Up and Cool Down

Add a warm-up to the start of your exercise and a cool-down at the end. Warm-up activities get your muscles and joints ready for the workout, which lowers your risk of getting hurt. A cool-down can include deep breathing and relaxation methods to help slow down your heart rate.

Keeping an eye on alignment

For chair yoga to be safe, you need to be in the right position. As you do each pose, pay close attention to your stance. Don't stretch or overextend any part of your body. Keep your back straight and your shoulders loose. Aligning yourself correctly not only keeps you safe, but it also makes each pose more effective.

Awareness of Breathing

One of the most important parts of yoga is breathing. Don't hold your breath during poses, and make sure you breathe deeply and mindfully. Breathing correctly helps you stay focused, keep your moves under control, and avoid injury or strain.

Speed and Intensity

Pay attention to your body and go at your own speed. If you're having trouble with a pose, either ease up or try a different version of it. Take care not to hurt or bother your body. It's important that the level of difficulty of your exercise is just right.

Changes for People with Different Abilities

Changes are an important part of chair yoga because they make it possible for people of all skills to do. If you need to, you can change the pose by adding yoga blocks, straps, or pillows. For instance, if it's hard to reach the floor, you can use a block to make it closer.

How to Avoid Common Mistakes

Be aware of mistakes that many people make, like locking your joints, slouching, or holding your breath. To avoid strain, keep your arms and knees slightly bent at all times. Don't round your back, and keep your spine long.

Pose for Balancing

If you want to get better at standing poses, keep your chair close by for support. To help you stay balanced, keep your breath steady and even. Change balanced poses as needed to keep people safe and comfortable.

Changing to Address Specific Health Issues

If you have certain health issues, like high blood pressure, vertigo, or heart issues, you should change how you do yoga. You might need to change or stay away from some poses. If you have vertigo, for example, stay away from or change poses that require quick moves or big changes in head position.

Keeping yourself hydrated

Drink water before, during, and after your workout. Water helps your body work at its best and can keep you from getting dizzy or lightheaded while you're working out.

Being Able to Stop

If at any point you feel dizzy, short of breath, or pain, stop right away. Rest, and if you need to, talk to a medical provider. Remember that yoga is about being aware of your body's limits and listening to it.

Final Thoughts

To do chair yoga safely, you need to know your physical limits, pick the right gear, pay attention to balance, go at your own pace, and make any necessary changes. If you follow these safety tips and pay attention to what your body needs, you can do chair yoga in a way that makes you feel good and helps you reach your weight loss and health goals.

PRAYER POSE

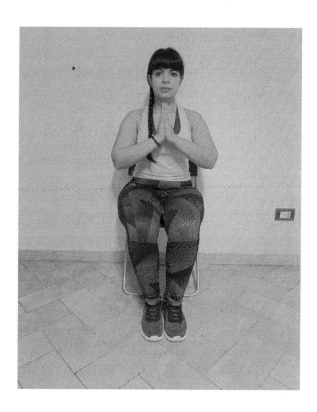

Instructions

1. Sit comfortably: Soak up some air in your chair before you start. Make sure your back is straight and your feet are flat on the ground, hip-width apart. If your feet don't reach the ground easily, put a block or some books under them to help them.

2. Loosen up your shoulders. Open your chest and roll your shoulders back and down to loosen them up. This helps you keep your back straight while still being relaxed.

3. Put your hands on your lap: To start, put your palms up and rest your hands on your thighs or lap. This will help you balance yourself.

4. Bring your palms together. Carefully bring your palms together in front of your chest, making sure your fingers stay pointed up. In many countries, the move looks like a prayer position.

5. Make sure your elbows are in line with your arms. This means that your elbows shouldn't be sagging or pushed up too high. Your wrists should be almost straight out from your body.

6. Gentle Pressure: Put a little pressure between your fingers, just enough to feel a connection but not so much that your hands or wrists get tense.

7. Close your eyes (if you want to) and focus on your breath and intention. You don't have to close your eyes to focus and concentrate. But if you want to, you can.

8. If you're deep breathing: Pay attention to your breathing while putting your hands in the prayer pose. Take a big breath in through your nose to fill your lungs, and then slowly let out all of your breath.

9. Make up your mind: You can make a goal for your practice while you're in this pose, or you can just use this time for meditation or quiet thought.

10. Letting Go of the Pose: After a few breaths or whenever you're ready, slowly take your hands off your lap and put them back on your lap.

11. Think about it: Think about any feelings or thoughts you had during the pose for a moment.

Tips and Changes:

- For Tight Shoulders: If bringing your palms together hurts because your shoulders are tight, change the pose by pressing only your fingertips together or keep your palms slightly apart.

- Adding mantras: Saying a prayer or affirmation quietly with each breath can help you get more out of the pose.

- It's good for transitions: This pose is often used to ease into or out of more busy poses or to take a moment to rest and think.

SIDE TWIST

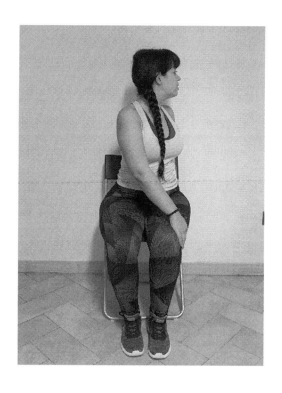 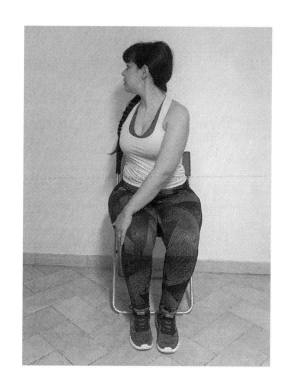

Instructions

1. Sit up straight: Place your feet flat on the floor, hip-width apart, and close to the front end of a chair. Keep your back straight.

2. Ground your feet: Make sure your feet are firmly on the ground or on blocks if they don't reach the floor.

3. Start the twist: as you let out a breath, turn your body to the right. Put your left hand on your right leg and your right hand on the chair's back.

4. Align Your Shoulders: Make sure your shoulders are level and loose.

5. Place of the gaze and the neck: If it's okay with you, turn your head to look over your right shoulder.

6. Keep your hips aligned: face forward with your hips and twist from the base of your back.

7. Take a few deep breaths and hold the twist for a few seconds. As you breathe in, lengthen your neck and twist deeper as you breathe out.

8. Go back to the middle: As you breathe in, slowly turn your body back to the front.

9. Do it again on the other side. To keep your balance, do the twist on the left side.

10. Sit up straight for a moment: Once you've done both sides, sit up straight and pay attention to how your body feels.

Tips and Changes:

1. Take it easy: start with a light twist and add more depth as you feel comfortable.

2. To make your neck feel better, don't turn your head; instead, keep it straight out from your chest.

As you breathe out, deepen the twist because your body automatically contracts during this phase.

4. Respect Limits: Don't force the twist; stay in the range of motion that feels good to you.

5. Use Props: If it's hard to reach the floor or keep your balance, use blocks or blankets to help.

SHOULDER CIRCLES

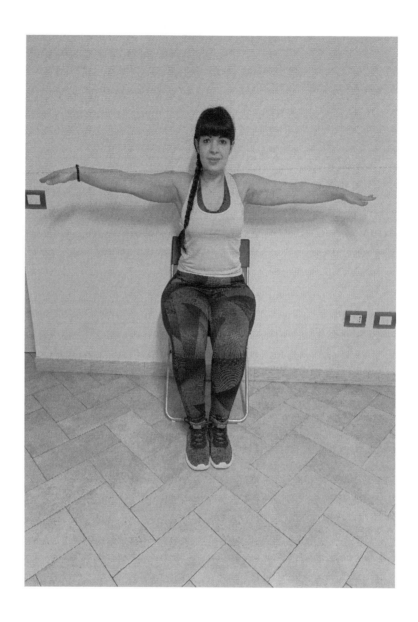

Instructions

1. Start by sitting up straight in a chair and placing your feet flat on the ground, hip-width apart. Put your hands on your legs.

2. Raise your arms up to shoulder height and out to the sides. Your hands should be facing down.

3. Turn your arms slowly so that your palms face up toward the sky. Then turn your arms back down.

4. Controlled Movement: Make sure the movement is smooth and steady, and focus on the shoulder rotation.

5. Repeat: Do this spinning motion as many times as it feels good to you.

Tips and Changes:

1. Keep your posture straight. Make sure your back stays straight and your shoulders are relaxed, not bent.

2. Breath Coordination: Time your breath with the action by breathing in as you turn your palms up and breathing out as you turn them down.

3. Adjust Range: If fully extending your arms hurts, bend your elbows a little or limit your range of motion.

4. Focus on Shoulders: Keep your attention on moving your shoulders and keep your other arms loose.

5. Alternate Movements: To change things up, you can rotate each arm in a different direction or try moving your wrists at the same time.

FOLD POSE

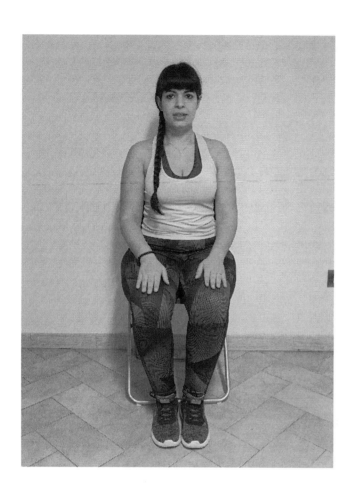 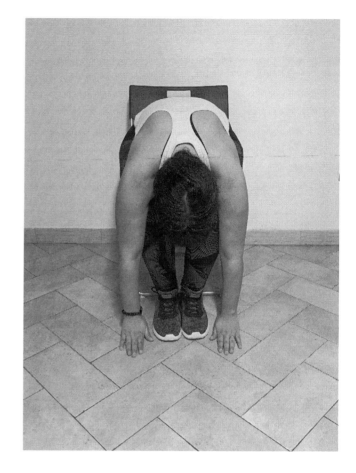

Instructions

1. Start by sitting on the side of a chair without arms. Place your feet flat on the floor, hip-width apart.

2. Align your spine: Sit up straight, which will make your spine longer.

3. To start the fold, hinge at the hips and bend forward while keeping your back straight.

4. Place your arms: Let your arms hang down toward the floor. They can be dangling, on the floor, or sitting on your shins.

5. Relax Your Neck: Don't tense up your head or neck.

6. Depth of Pose: Fold in as far as you can easily.

7. Hold Pose: Stay in the fold for a few breaths, slowly getting deeper with each exhale.

8. When you come out, slowly roll up to a sitting position, making sure your head comes up last.

Tips and Changes:

- Being Gentle for Back Problems: If you have back pain or tight legs, be gentle. Just fold it as far as it feels good.
- Yoga blocks or a cushion can help you if you can't reach the floor.
- For knee comfort, bend your knees a little or put a towel rolled up under them if you need to.
- Pay attention to your breathing. Use your breath to help you relax and go deeper into the pose.

LOW LUNGE

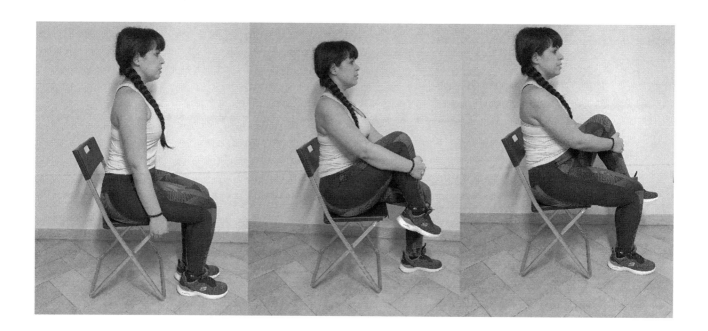

Instructions

1. As you sit easily in chair,, stretch your back and let your shoulders drop. Make sure you're sitting easily and that your feet are flat on the ground.

2. Take a deep breath in and lift your right leg while bending your knees. Put your hands below your right thigh to support it.

3. As you let out your breath, flex your right ankle and bring your thigh up to your chest. Keep your back straight and point your toes down. Bring your knee close to your chest.

4. Hold this pose for at least four to six breaths. Pay attention to how the hips, lower back, core, and pelvic floor muscles stretch.

5. As you let out a breath, let go of the leg and sit back with both feet on the floor.

6. If you need to, adjust the hips. Then take a deep breath in and lift your left leg up, holding it below your thighs with your hand.

7. As you let out a breath, press your thighs close to your chest. Hold for four to six breaths, then let go and rest. To get better, do the same thing again and again.

Tips and Changes:

- For hip comfort, change how far forward your foot is from the ground or how far back your back leg is stretched out.
- Support for Balance: If it's hard for you to keep your balance, put your hands on your forward knee or grab the chair's sides.
- Knee Safety: To protect your knee joint, make sure your forward knee is right above your ankle and not sticking out past your toes.
- Gentle Movement: To stay balanced, enter and leave the pose slowly. Do not move quickly.

COBRA POSE

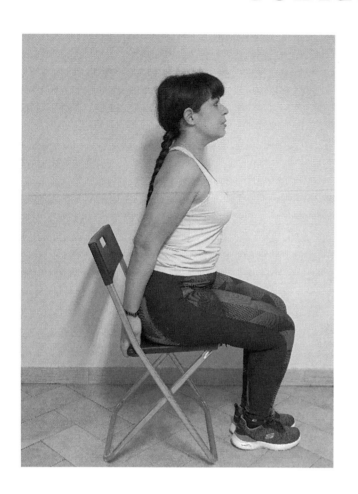 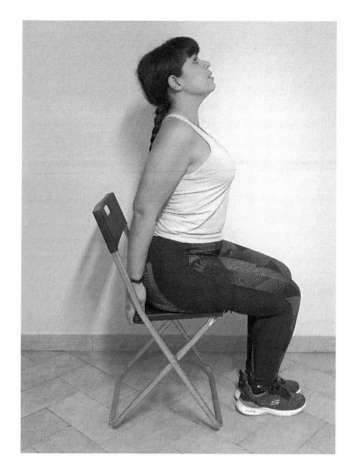

Instructions

1. Sit on the edge of a chair with your feet flat on the floor and your hips far apart.

2. Put your hands on the back of your waist or the small of your back.

3. Lengthen Spine: Take a deep breath in and slowly straighten your back while sitting up straight.

4. When you let your breath out, slowly arch your back, pushing your chest forward and up and pulling your shoulder blades together. If it feels good, tilt your head back a little.

5. Hold Pose: Stay in this pose for a few breaths, focused on the gentle stretch in your back and how it opens up your chest.

6. Release: Take a deep breath in and slowly move your neck back to a neutral position.

Tips and Changes:

- Intensity Adjustment: You can change how hard the backbend is to suit your needs. The stretch shouldn't hurt, it should be soft.

- Neck Care: Keep your neck in a relaxed position and don't strain it, especially when you tilt your head back.

- Use of Props: If you need extra support for your lower back, use a cushion.

- Focus on Breathing: Breathe easily during the pose to help you relax and feel your chest and back open up.

ONE-LEGGED SEATED FORWARD BEND

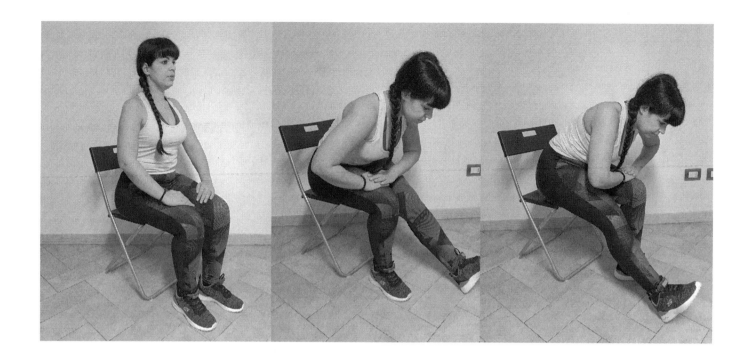

Instructions

1. To begin, sit in a chair with your feet flat on the ground, hip-width apart.

2. "Extend One Leg": Keep the heel of one leg on the ground and the toes looking up as you extend it forward. One of the feet stays flat on the ground.

3. Align Your Spine: Sit up straight, which will make your spine longer. Take deep breaths.

4. To start the bend, let out a breath and slightly hinge at the hips, leaning forward toward the leg that is stretched out. Do not bend over.

5. Stand with your hands together and reach them toward the leg that is outstretched. Based on how flexible you are, you can rest them on your shin, ankle, or foot.

6. Hold the Pose: Stay in the pose for a few breaths, letting out more air with each exhale.

7. Release: Take a deep breath in and slowly sit back up.

Eighth, "Switch Legs." Do the same thing again with the other leg stretched out.

Tips and Changes:

- Gentle Stretch: Don't stretch too far. The goal is for the back of the leg that is stretched out and your lower back to feel a light stretch.

- Don't lock your knees. If it feels better, keep the knee of the leg you're extending slightly bent.

- Handle Props: If it's hard to reach your foot, wrap a yoga strap or a towel around it to keep the stretch going without hurting.

- Maintain Posture: Don't think about how far you can reach, just keep your back straight. This keeps the muscles from straining and makes sure the stretch goes to the right places.

- Breathe Smoothly: Move in sync with your breath, making the bend deeper when you breathe out.

PIGEON STRETCH

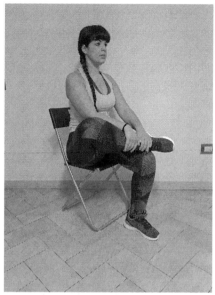 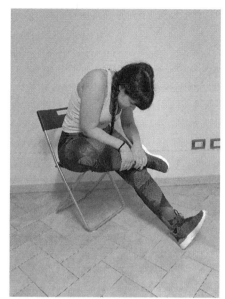

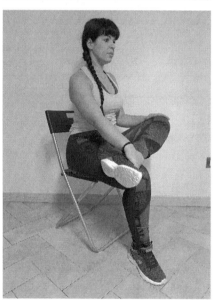 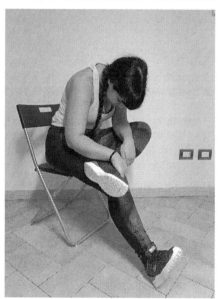

Instructions

1. If you're sitting, put your feet flat on the floor and your back straight.

2. Lift your right leg up and put your right ankle on your left thigh, just above the knee. Let your right knee hang open to the side and stay loose.

3. Align Your Spine: Sit up straight, which will make your spine longer. Take a big breath.

4. To start the stretch, let out a breath and lean forward slowly from your hips while keeping your back straight. Increase the stretch until it feels good.

5. Hold the Pose: Stay in this position for a few breaths, letting out more air with each exhale.

6. Let go: slowly stand up straight again and lower your right leg.

7. Switch Legs: Stretch your left leg again.

Tips and Changes:

- Be Gentle: If you feel any pain, especially in the knee or hip of the bent leg, either ease up on the stretch or put a cushion under your thigh to cushion it.

- Don't Put Pressure on Knee: Make sure your ankle is higher than your knee to keep from putting direct pressure on the knee joint.

- Use of Hands: You can add extra support with your hands on the bent leg to make the stretch deeper or on the chair to keep your balance.

- Maintain Alignment: To make sure you're in the right position, keep your shoulders and hips squared forward.

- Mind Your Breath: Take deep breaths to help you relax and slowly deepen the stretch. Taking slow, deep breaths can help ease stress.

HANDS UP

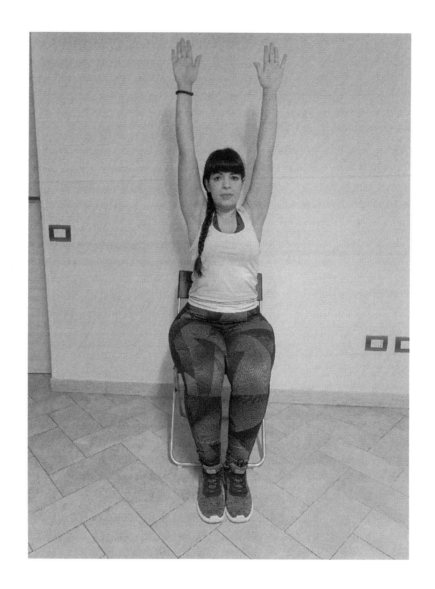

Instructions

1. Sit down first: Place your feet flat on the floor, hip-width apart, and sit down in a chair. Make sure your back is straight.

2. Place your arms in a certain way: put your hands on your legs.

3. Breathe in and lift your arms: Lift your arms slowly out to the sides and then up over your head as you breathe in. Depending on how flexible your shoulders are, your palms can face each other or touch.

4. Lengthen Your Spine: As you lift your arms, focus on making your spine longer by stretching up from the top of your head.

5. Stay in the pose by holding your arms up and taking deep breaths. Do not tense your shoulders and keep them away from your ears.

6. Let go: Let out a breath and slowly bring your arms back to your sides, putting your hands back on your legs.

Tips and Changes:

- Comfortable Shoulders: If it hurts to lift your arms all the way up, just lift them to a level that works for you. You'll get a good stretch even at half-mast.

- How to Use Props: If your shoulders don't move easily, you could hold a strap or towel between your hands to help keep your arms straight.

- Pay attention to your posture: keep your back straight and don't twist your lower back as you lift your arms.

- Breathing Coordination: Match your breath to your action by breathing in as you lift your arms and breathing out as you lower them.

- Neck Alignment: Make sure your neck stays straight, in line with your spine, and doesn't tilt back.

HIGH LUNGE

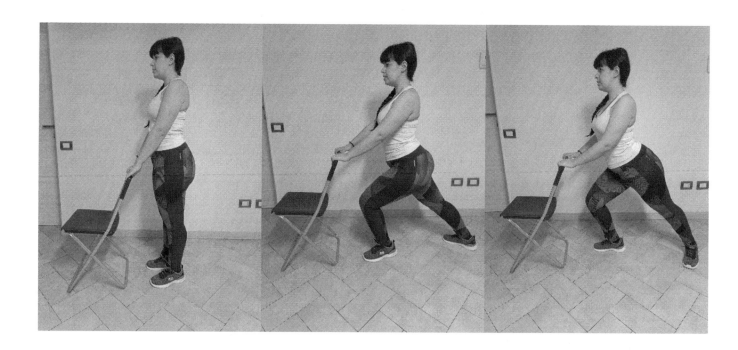

Instructions

1. Sit cross-legged on the edge of a chair without arms. Keep your feet flat on the floor, hip-width apart.

2. Slide your right foot forward and put it firmly on the ground with your knee bent 90 degrees. Your thigh should be flat on the ground.

3. Stretch Back Leg: Keep the ball of your left foot on the ground and stretch your left leg back. The tip of your foot should be off the ground and your leg should be straight.

4. Align Your Torso: Stand up straight and tall, and keep your back straight. For a better stretch and more balance, put your hands on your right thigh or lift them above your head.

5. Straighten your hips so they are square to the front of the chair.

6. Take a few deep breaths and stay in this pose for a few seconds. Focus on the stretch in your left hip flexor and the strength in your right leg.

7. Change Side: Let go of the pose gently, and then do it again with your left foot forward and your right leg stretched back.

Tips and Changes:

- Equal: If it's hard to keep your balance, put your hands on your forward knee or hold on to the chair.

- Safety for the Knees: Make sure that the knee of the leg you're putting forward is right above your ankle and doesn't go past your toes.

- Gentle Movement: Come into and out of the pose slowly to keep your balance and avoid moving quickly.

- Adjust the Stretch: Change the distance of your forward foot and the length of your back leg to change how hard the stretch is in your hip flexor.

WARRIOR POSE

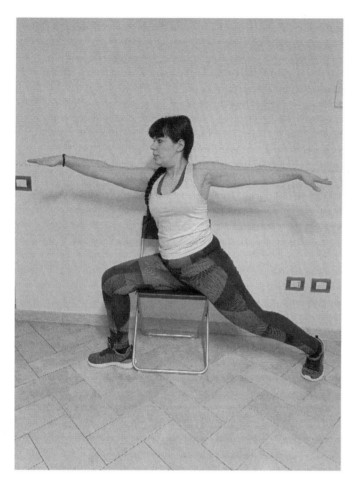 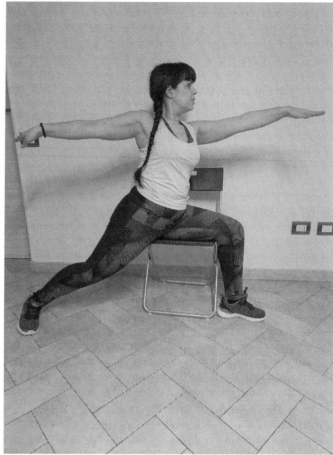

Instructions

1. Sit down first: Sit on the edge of a chair that doesn't have arms. Lay your feet flat on the ground, about hip-width apart.

2. Put the legs in place: Move your left foot in a little and your right foot out 90 degrees. Lay your left leg back and rest the ball of your foot on the ground. Make sure the leg stays straight.

3. Line up your hips: Make sure your hips are square to the front of the chair. The floor should be level with your right thigh.

4. Raise your arms: Hold your arms out to the sides, shoulder-width apart, and straight out from your body. Right arm should be over right leg, and left arm should be stretched out behind you.

5. Look ahead: Look over your right hand with your head turned. Not too high or too low. Keep your chest open.

6. Take a few deep breaths and stay in this pose for a few seconds. Focus on how strong your arms are and how your legs feel stretched.

7. Switch Sides: Let go of the pose gently and do it again on the other side, this time with your right leg stretched back and your left foot turned out.

Tips and Changes:

- Arm Placement: If fully raising your arms hurts, keep them at a lower level or rest your hands on your hips.

- For knee safety, make sure your forward knee is right above your ankle and doesn't go past your toes.

- Remember to keep your hips square to the front. Change where your back leg is placed to keep your body in the right position.

- Pay attention to your posture: keep your back straight and use your core muscles to stay stable.

- As you raise your arms and lower them, make sure your breath goes with the pose. For example, breathe in as you raise your arms and breathe out as you lower them.

HUMBLE WARRIOR POSE

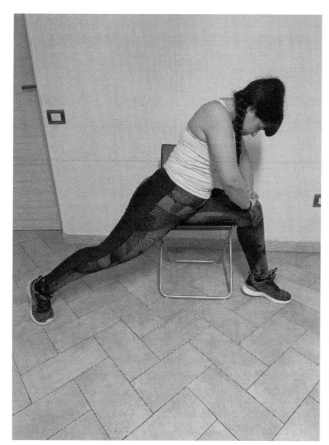 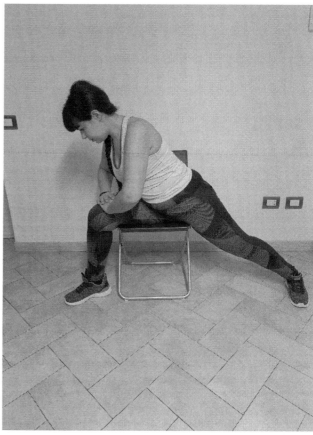

Instructions

1. Start by sitting on the tip of a chair without arms. Keep your feet flat on the floor and your hip-width apart.

2. Put the legs in place: Stretch your left leg back and put the ball of your left foot on the ground. Turn your right foot out 90 degrees. The floor should be level with the right thigh.

3. Line up your hips: Make sure your hips are square to the front of the chair.

4. Join your fingers together: Put your hands behind your back and cross your fingers.

5. Lean forward, take a deep breath in, and stretch out your back. Lean forward from your hips over your right leg as you let out your breath. As you lift your hands off of your back and up toward the sky, lower your chest toward your right knee.

6. Bow Your Head: Lower your head and look at the ground or your right foot.

7. Hold the Pose: Stay in this forward bend for a few breaths, letting your shoulders and right thigh stretch.

8. Get up: As you breathe in, slowly lift your body back up while letting go of your hands.

9. Turn Sides: On the left side, do the pose again with your right leg stretched back and your left foot turned out.

Tips and Changes:

- Comfortable Shoulders: If it hurts to cross your fingers behind your back, put a strap or towel between your hands to make the stretch less severe.

- Maintain Balance: To keep your balance as you lean forward, focus on grounding through your sitting position.

- Soft Neck: When you bow your head, don't strain your neck. Instead, keep it loose.

- Intensity Adjustment: Change how hard the forward bend is for you based on how comfortable it is. It's more important to keep your back straight than to get deeper into the pose.

- Breathing: During the pose, breathe easily, and with each exhale, gently bend forward.

SUN BREATHS

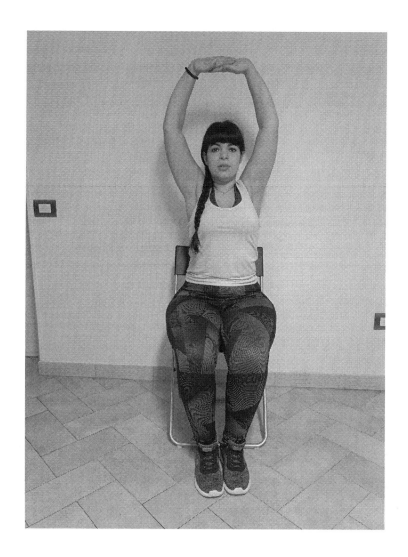

Instructions

1. Sit down in a chair that is comfortable for you, preferably one without arms. Place your feet flat on the floor and hip-width apart.

2. First Position of the Hands: Put your palms facing up and rest your hands on your legs or lap.

3. Breathe in and lift your arms: As you slowly breathe in, lift your arms out to the sides and then up over your head. As long as your shoulders are loose, your palms can face each other or touch at the top.

4. Let out energy and lower your arms: As you let your breath out, bring your arms back to your sides and then to your lap to finish the circle.

5. Coordinate with Breath: Do this moving movement a few times, making sure that your arm movements match your breath. For example, breathe in as you lift your arms and breathe out as you lower them.

6. Pay attention to your movement: Let your movement be smooth and graceful, matching the beat of your breath.

Tips and Changes:

- Area of Motion: You can change the range until it feels good if raising your arms fully overhead hurts.

- How to Use Props: If your shoulders don't move easily, you might want to hold a strap between your hands to keep them in place.

- Maintain Posture: When your arms are lifted, keep your back straight and don't arch it too much.

- Neck Alignment: Make sure your neck stays straight and doesn't pull forward or backward.

- Mindful Breathing: Focus on taking deep, even breaths to help you relax and feel more energized from the movement.

NECK ROLLS

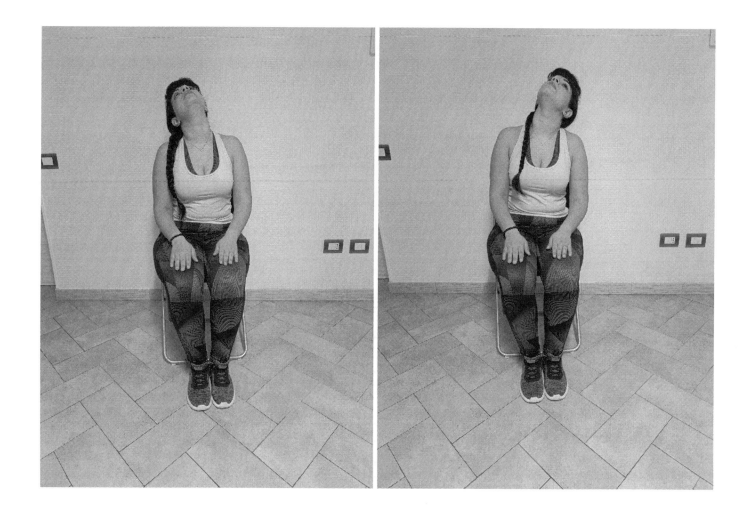

Instructions

1. Sit down first: Place your feet flat on the floor, hip-width apart, and sit down in a chair. Keep your shoulders loose and your back straight.

2. Start with your head in a neutral pose and your eyes facing forward.

3. Bring your chin down to your chest slowly to start the roll. You should feel a stretch in the back of your neck.

4. Side stretch: Roll your head slowly to the right shoulder until your ear is close to the shoulder.

5. Do the "Backward Roll." Keep gently rolling your head backward, but only as far as it feels good and doesn't put too much pressure on your neck.

6. Finish the Circle. Roll your left shoulder over to your right shoulder and then bring your chin back to your chest.

7. Repeat: Do this move in a circle a few times, then turn it around.

Tips and Changes:

- Movements that are slow: Move your head slowly and gently so you don't get dizzy or strain your neck.

- Area of Motion: You should only roll your head back as far as feels good. If it makes you feel bad or puts stress on your neck, move the roll forward.

- Maintain Good Posture: To avoid stress, keep your shoulders loose and your back straight during the activity.

- Breathe Deeply: Move in time with your breath, taking deep breaths in and out.

- Avoid Full Circles If You Can: If full neck rolls hurt, you can change the shape of the move so that your chin is to your chest as you move from one shoulder to the other.

NECK ROLLS: DOWN AND UP

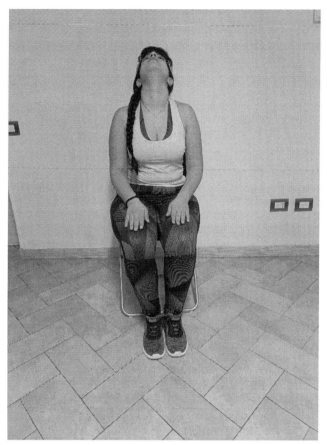 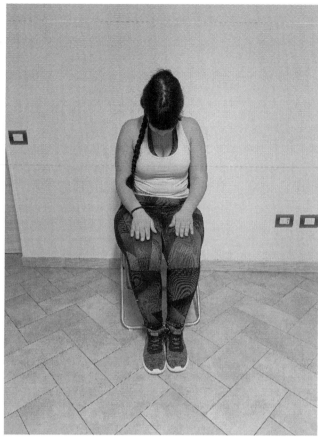

Instructions

1. Sit down first: Place your feet flat on the floor, hip-width apart, and sit in a chair. Keep your shoulders loose and your back straight.

2. Start with your head in a neutral pose and your eyes facing forward.

3. Chin to Chest: Lower your chin slowly toward your chest until you feel a stretch in the back of your neck.

4. Roll Downward: Bring your right ear to your right shoulder as you slowly roll your head down to the right.

5. To reverse the roll, slowly roll your head back to a position where your chin is against your chest.

6. Roll to the Other Side: Bring your left ear to your left shoulder and roll to the left side again.

7. Finish the Cycle: Go back to the chin-to-chest pose.

8. Say it again: Keep moving in this half-circle pattern for a few rounds.

Tips and Changes:

- Gentle Shakes: If you don't want to feel pain or dizziness, move your head slowly and gently.

- Range is limited: Reduce the range of motion to a level that feels good if full downward rolls make you feel bad.

- Maintain Posture: To avoid injury, keep your back straight and shoulders loose.

- Breathing: Move in sync with your breath; breathe in when you're in the neutral position and breathe out when you roll your neck.

- Focus on Stretch: Pay attention to how your neck muscles are stretching and don't make any forced moves.

SIDE STRETCH

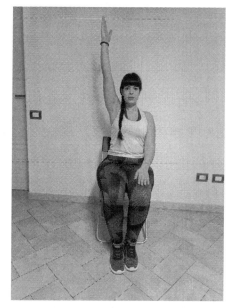
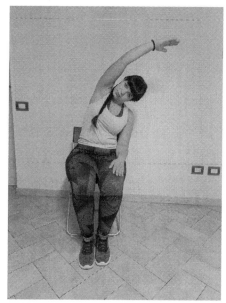
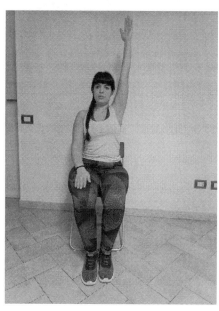
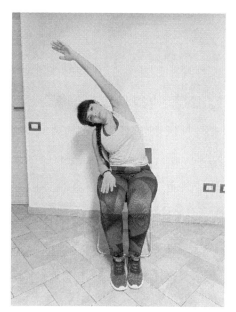

Instructions

1. Sit down first: Place your feet flat on the floor, hip-width apart, and sit down in a chair. Hold your shoulders back and your back straight.

2. Place your hands on your legs or lap for the first time.

3. Raise One Arm: Take a deep breath in and lift your right arm up toward the sky, making sure your shoulder stays loose.

4. Start the side stretch: Stretch the right side of your body by leaning your chest to the left as you let out your breath. Stretch out your right arm and rest your left hand on your thigh or the side of the chair to support yourself.

5. Stay in alignment: Don't bend forward or backward, and keep your hips firmly on the chair. It's best to stretch along the side of your neck.

6. Hold the Pose: Stay in this side stretch for a few breaths and feel your ribs and side of your waist get bigger.

7. Return to Center: Take a deep breath in as you stand up straight with your right arm dropped.

8. Do It Again on the Other Side: Lift your left arm and lean to the right to do the stretch again on the left side.

Tips and Changes:

- Arm Placement: Your hand can stay on your hip or be stretched out at a lower angle if lifting it above your head hurts.
- Soft Stretch: Be careful not to stretch too far. It shouldn't hurt or feel awkward to move.
- Comfort for the Neck: Make sure your neck is loose and in line with your spine. Do not pull it to the side.
- Breath Coordination: Pull in your breath to make the stretch deeper, and let out your breath to slowly lengthen the stretch.
- Core Engagement: Lightly engage your core muscles to help support you and make the stretch better.

CAT COW

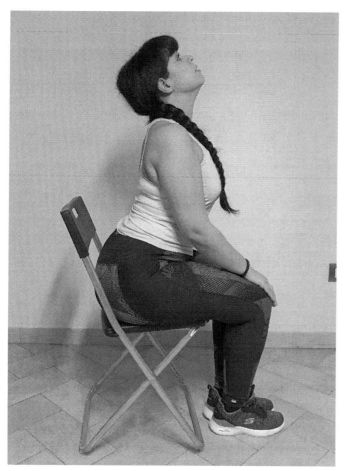 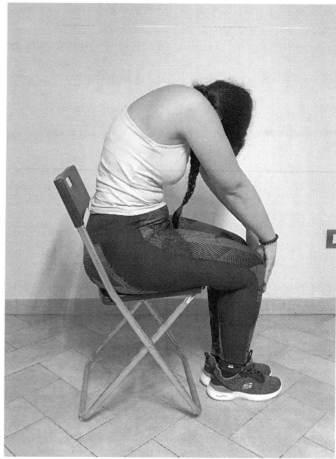

Instructions

1. Sit down first: Place your feet flat on the floor, hip-width apart, and sit on the edge of a chair. Kneel down and put your hands on them.

2. Inhale into the cow pose: As you breathe in, arch your back, push your chest forward, and tilt your hips back. Look a little higher with your eyes and pull your shoulders back.

3. Cat Pose (Do Not Inhale): When you let your breath out, round your back, tuck your hips under, and bring your chin to your chest. Pull your belly button in toward your spine slowly, and round your shoulders forward.

4. Flow from one pose to the next: Keep moving easily from the Cow Pose to the Cat Pose on inhales and exhales, making a rhythmic movement.

5. Do this process over and over again, following the rhythm of your breath each time.

Tips and Changes:

- Gentle Movement:Move in a way that feels good, especially if you have back problems.
- Take a look at the spine: Make sure that your spine is where the action starts. Picture each spine moving one after the other.
- Attention to Breathing: Make sure your actions and breathing go together smoothly for a smooth flow.
- Neck Care: Make sure your neck is straight with your spine and don't strain it too much when you look up or tuck your chin in.
- Engage Core: Flex your abs gently to support your back, especially when you round your back in the Cat Pose.

LEG EXTENSIONS (ASSISTED)

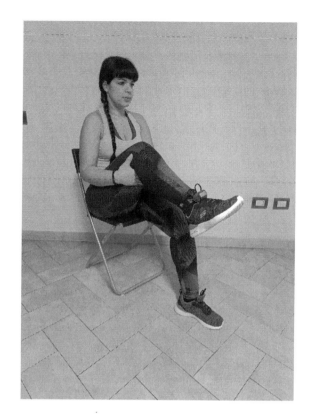 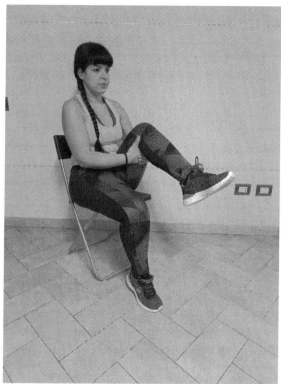

Instructions

1. Sit down first: Place your feet flat on the floor, hip-width apart, and sit in a chair. A better way to get around is to sit close to the edge of the chair.

2. Start by putting your hands on the sides of the chair to support yourself. Keep your back straight and your shoulders loose.

3. Slowly put your right leg out in front of you, making sure the foot stays bent and the leg is as straight as it can be.

4. Raise Leg: Lift the leg that is outstretched to a reasonable height. This will work the muscles in your thighs.

5. Hold the Pose. Stay in this stretched-out pose for a few seconds, focusing on how your leg muscles feel strong and stretched.

6. Lower Leg: Carefully lower your leg back to where it started.

7. Do it again with the other leg: move your left leg in the same way.

8. Switch the legs: Switch between legs again and again for a few reps.

Tips and Changes:

- Moves that are controlled: To keep muscles from jerking or stretching, make sure each movement is steady and under control.

- Use of Strap: If it's hard to lift your leg, put a yoga strap or towel under your foot to help you extend.

- Change Height: Lift your leg up as high as it feels good. Not how high you can lift, but how well you can control your movements and use your muscles.

- Breathing: Time your breath with the movement by breathing in as you lift the leg and breathing out as you lower it.

- Keep Core Engaged: To make the exercise more stable, lightly engage your core muscles as you do it.

FOOT FLEXING

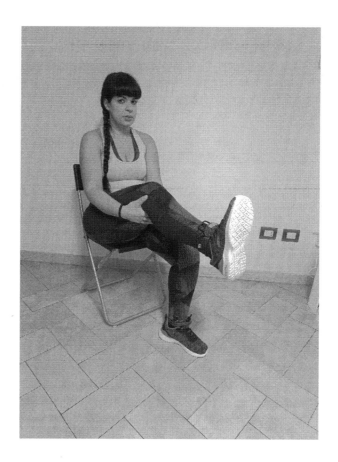

Instructions

1. Put your feet flat on the ground about hip-width apart and sit in a chair. Make sure your shoulders are loose and your back is straight.

2. In the "Initial Position," put your hands on your legs or hold on to the chair's sides to stay steady.

3. Flex Forward: Bring one leg forward and straight out from your body. Pull your toes toward your shin as you bend your foot. You can feel your leg and the bottom of your foot getting stretched.

4. Hold the Stretch. Keep your leg bent for a few seconds and focus on the stretch in your lower leg.

5. Point your toes away from you. This will stretch the top of your foot and shin.

6. Hold Again: Stay in this position for a few seconds.

7. Alternate Feet: Bring your other foot down to the ground and do the same steps with your other foot.

8. Say it again: Switching between bending and pointing each foot several times will help you get better.

Tips and Changes:

- Gentle Movements: Move your feet slowly and steadily, and don't make any sudden movements.

- Area of Motion: Just bend and point your foot as far as it feels good. It shouldn't hurt to move around.

- Using Your Hands: To make the stretch stronger, you can lightly press on your toes while your foot is bent.

- Maintain Posture: Don't lean back as you extend your leg; instead, keep your neck straight.

- Breathing: Time your action with your breathing by breathing in when you bend and out when you point.

CACTUS ARMS

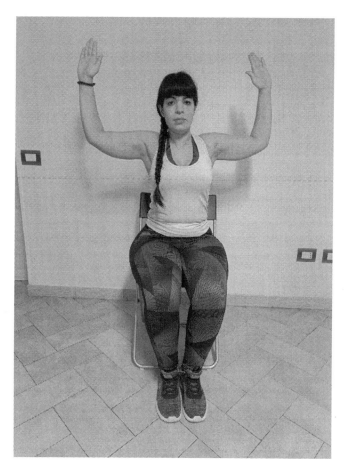 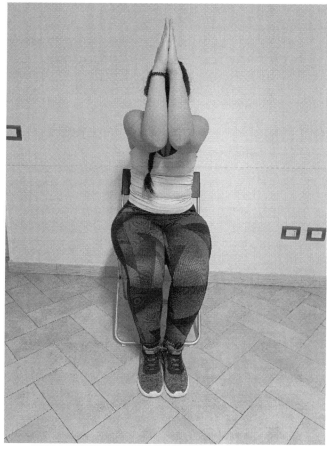

Instructions

1. Sit down first: Place your feet flat on the floor, hip-width apart, and sit down in a chair. Hold your shoulders back and your back straight.

2. Raise your arms: Lift your arms out to the sides until they are at shoulder height. Bend your elbows so that they are at a 90-degree angle. Your upper arms should be straight out from your body.

3. For the "cactus shape," turn your hands outward and spread your fingers apart. When you bend your elbows and face your hands forward, your arms should look like a cactus.

4. "Open the chest" Pull your arms back slowly and squeeze your shoulder blades together. This makes your chest bigger.

5. Hold the Pose: Stay in this position for a few breaths, focused on how your chest opens up and your shoulders stretch.

6. Relax your arms and put them back in your lap or at your sides.

Tips and Changes:

- Comfortable Shoulders: If you're having trouble with your shoulders, move your arms forward a little to fix the position.

- Aligning the Neck: Don't stretch your neck backwards; instead, keep it loose and in line with your spine.

- Breath Coordination: Inhale as you open your chest and exhale as you relax. Make sure your breath goes with the action.

- Engage Core: Use your abs lightly to keep your back straight and your spine supported.

- Variation in Flexibility: If you're more flexible, you can move your arms back slowly to make the stretch deeper, but only as far as it feels good.

SAGE TWIST

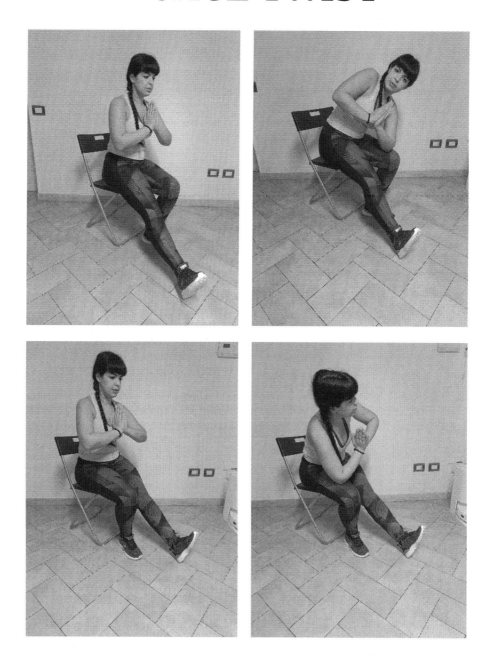

Instructions

1. Sit down first: Sit in a chair that is comfortable for you and doesn't have arms. Place your feet flat on the floor, hip-width apart. Keep your back straight and your shoulders back.

2. Start by putting your left hand on your right knee and your right hand behind you on the chair's seat or backrest to support yourself.

3. Start the twist: Take a deep breath in and stretch out your back. As you let out your breath, slowly turn your body to the right. Start turning at the base of your spine and work your way up to your neck.

4. Look over your right shoulder. If it feels good, turn your head to look over your right shoulder, which will make the twist stronger.

5. "Hold the Pose": Keep the twist for a few breaths, breathing in to stretch the spine and breathing out to make the twist deeper.

6. "Return to Center": Take a deep breath in and slowly move back to the front while letting go of the twist.

7. Do it again on the other side: Change hands and put your left hand behind you and your right hand on your left knee. Then do the twist again on the left side.

Tips and Changes:

- Be careful when moving: Don't force or stretch yourself as you move into the twist. It should be easy and smooth to move.
- Taking Care of Your Neck: Make sure your neck is straight with your spine. You should only turn your head as far as it feels good.
- Use of Arms: Use your arms to help strengthen the twist slowly, but don't use too much force.
- Spine Alignment: During the twist, try to keep your back straight and tall, and don't slouch or collapse.
- Breathing: Time your breath with the movement by breathing in to stretch and out to twist.

REVOLVED POSE

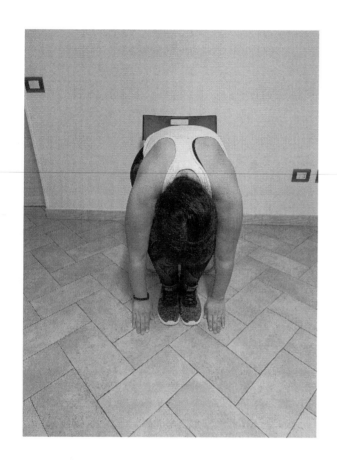 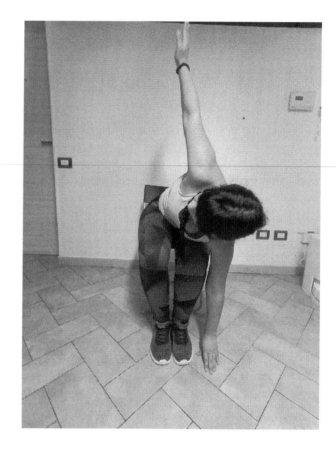

Instructions

1. Place your feet flat on the floor, hip-width apart, and sit in a chair that doesn't have arms. Make sure your back is straight when you sit up.

2. Get ready to twist: put your left hand on your right knee and your right hand on the chair next to you or on the bench to support yourself.

3. Start the Twist: Take a deep breath in and stretch out your back. As you let out your breath, slowly turn to the right. Start twisting at the base of your spine and work your way up through your middle and upper back.

4. Deepen the Twist: If it feels good, use your left hand on your right knee as support to deepen the twist with each exhale.

5. Neck and head: You can turn your head to look over your right shoulder if you want to, but only as far as it feels good.

6. Stick with the pose: Hold the twist for a few breaths, focused on keeping your back straight.

7. Go back to the middle: As you breathe in, slowly move back to the front and let go of the twist.

8. Do it again on the other side. This time, put your right hand on your left knee and twist to the left.

Tips and Changes:

- Gentle Approach: Take your time and move slowly into the twist. If you already have back problems, don't push or force yourself.
- Be Smart About Your Arms: Use your arms for support and power, but don't twist too hard.
- Align Your Spine: Don't move forward or backward, and keep your spine straight.
- Coordination for Breathing: To lengthen the spine, breathe in, and to strengthen the twist, breathe out. This makes it easier to move and keeps you from straining.
- Neck Comfort: Make sure your neck is in a good place. When you turn your head, don't strain it too much. Keep it straight along with the rest of your back.

BOAT

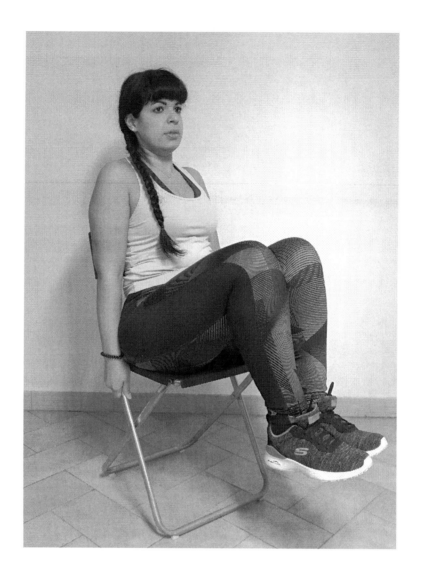

Instructions

1. Place your feet flat on the floor, hip-width apart, and bend your knees. Sit on the edge of a chair. For balance, hold on to the chair's sides.

2. Lean Back Slightly: Keep your chest up and your back straight as you lean back a little. Use the muscles in your middle.

3. Lift Your Legs: Lift your feet off the ground and line up your shins with the floor. If you can, put your legs straight out in front of you so that your body forms a "V."

4. Arm Position: If you feel stable, take your hands off the chair and straighten your arms out in front of you.

5. "Balance and Hold": Stay in this pose for a few breaths while you balance on your sit bones. Don't bend over, and keep your core tight.

6. Let go: Lower your feet slowly back to the floor and let go of your arms.

Tips and Changes:

- Begin by bending your knees: If it's hard for you to fully extend your legs, bend your knees. Pay attention to keeping your balance and using your core.

- Alignment of the spine: Your back will thank you if you keep your neck straight. Do not make your shoulders round.

- Breathing: Take slow, even breaths throughout the pose. Taking deep, steady breaths will help you stay balanced.

- Gradual Progression: As your core strength and balance get better, slowly work your way up to raising your legs.

- Use of Arms: If you need more support, keep your hands on the sides of the chair.

LEG RAISES

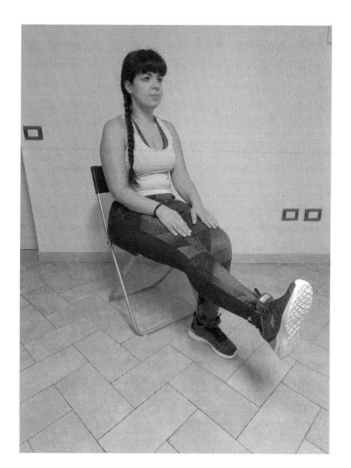 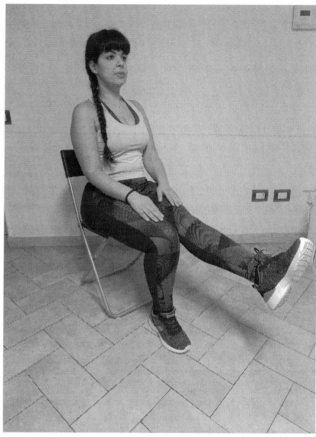

Instructions

1. Place your feet flat on the floor, hip-width apart, and sit in a chair that doesn't have arms. A better way to get around is to sit close to the edge of the chair.

2. Alignment of the spine: To stay balanced and strong, keep your back straight and hold on to the chair's sides.

3. As you slowly lift your right leg off the ground, try to keep it straight. Raise it until it's at a good height for you.

4. Keep your leg higher for a few seconds to work the muscles in your thigh.

5. Carefully lower your leg back to where it started.

6. Move your left leg in the same way.

7. Keep switching between your right and left legs for a few more reps.

Tips and Changes:

- Controlled Movement: Make sure that you can control each lift. To avoid strain, don't move in rapid ways.

- Coordinating your breath: Take a deep breath in as you lift your leg and let it go as you lower it. This helps you stay focused and in sync.

- Area of Motion: Lift your leg up as high as it feels good. The goal is on moving with control, not on height.

- Core Engagement: While lifting your leg, use your core muscles to help keep you stable and give your lower back extra support.

- Progress Gradually: As your strength grows, slowly increase the number of reps or the height of the leg raises.

CHAIR SQUATS

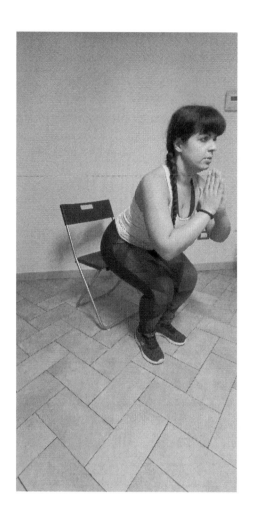

Instructions

1. Stand up straight. Put your feet hip-width apart and point your toes forward in front of a chair. You should have the chair behind you.

2. Alignment of the spine: Keep your shoulders loose and your back straight. For balance, put your arms out in front of you or keep them at your sides.

3. Start the squat. Put your weight back on your feet and bend your knees as if you were going to sit down.

4. Raise Your Hands: Bring your body down slowly toward the chair. Stand up straight and lift your chest.

5. Touch and Lift: Keep your bottom close to the chair but don't sit down all the way. Right away, push through your heels to get back up.

6. Repeat: Do this move over and over again, making sure to keep your control and good form the whole time.

Tips and Changes:

- Controlled Motion: Make sure the motion is slow and steady. Do not fall asleep in the chair.

- Alignment of the Knees: Make sure your knees are straight over your feet and don't go past your toes.

- To improve your breath coordination, breathe in as you lower yourself and breathe out as you stand up.

- Squat Depth: Change the depth to suit your strength and comfort. The exercise will help you even if you don't go very low.

- Use of Arms: If you need to, stretch out your arms to help you stay balanced. You can make it harder by crossing your arms over your chest as you get stronger.

CALF RAISES

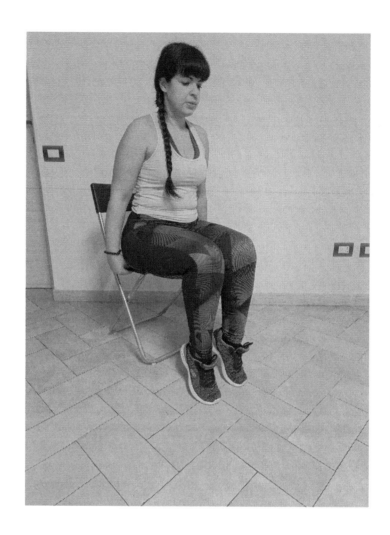

Instructions

1. Place your feet flat on the floor, hip-width apart, and sit in a chair. Keep your shoulders loose and your back straight.

2. Put your feet flat on the ground and make sure your ankles are in line with your knees.

3. To lift your heels off the ground and lift your legs, push down through the balls of your feet.

4. Keep your legs higher for a few seconds, working the muscles in your calves.

5. Put your heels back on the floor slowly.

6. Do this move over and over again while keeping your form smooth and controlled.

Tips and Changes:

- Controlled Movement: To get the most out of your muscles, lift and lower slowly and steadily.

- Spine Alignment: Stand up straight during the whole workout and don't lean forward.

- Taking a breath: Make sure your breath goes with the movement. Breathe in as you lift your feet and breathe out as you lower them.

- Positioning of the Feet: When you don't lift your feet, make sure they stay flat and evenly pressed against the floor. Do not roll to the outside or inside edges of your feet.

- Progress: As your power grows, you can either do more reps or add ankle weights to meet more resistance.

ALTERNATIVE CALF RAISES

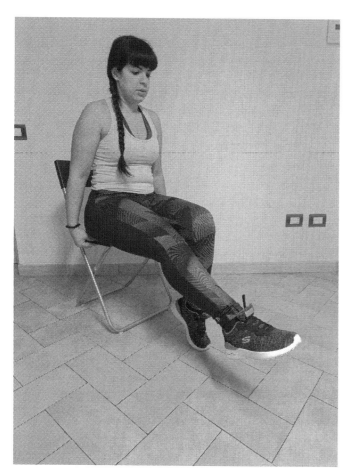 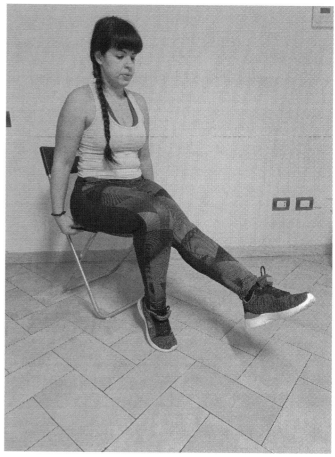

Instructions

1. Start by sitting down. Place your feet flat on the floor, hip-width apart, and sit on a chair. Make sure your shoulders are loose and your back straight.

2. Heel Lifts: Keep your toes and balls of your feet on the ground and lift your heels off the floor. As you lift your feet, work your calf muscles.

3. After putting your heels back on the floor, lift your toes and the balls of your feet and put your weight on your heels. The muscles in the front of your shins will get stronger.

4. Move your feet back and forth between lifting your heels and your toes, making a rocking motion with your feet.

5. Keep doing this alternating rhythm over and over, making sure to keep your movement smooth and controlled.

Tips and Changes:

- Controlled Motion: Don't worry about speed; instead, focus on slow, deliberate actions.

- Posture: During the practice, keep your back straight. Do not move forward.

- To keep a steady rhythm, breathe in during one part of the move (heels or toes) and out during the other.

- Flexibility in the ankles: This movement also helps make your ankles more flexible. If there is a part of the movement that is harder, work on it more slowly for a little while longer.

- Progress: As your strength and flexibility improve, you can either do more reps or add ankle weights to make the exercise harder.

MOUNTAIN POSE ONE LEG

BACKLIFT

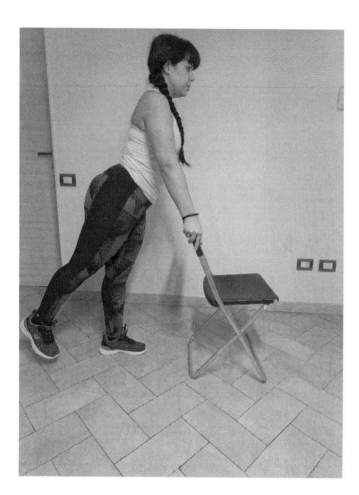 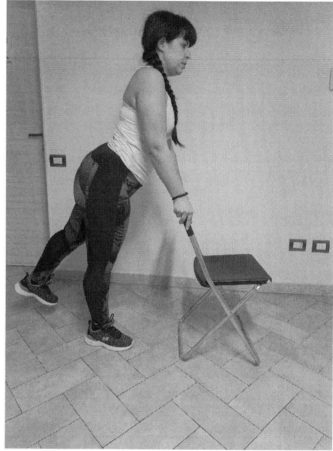

Instructions

1. Sit down first: Place your feet flat on the floor, hip-width apart, and sit in a chair that doesn't have arms. Make sure your shoulders are loose and your back straight.

2. Get Stable: To get stable, press your sitting bones into the seat and use your core muscles to support yourself.

3. Raise One Leg: Keep your right leg as straight as possible as you slowly lift and stretch it behind you. It's important that the movement comes from your hips and not from moving forward.

4. Hold the Pose: Keep your leg raised for a few seconds, making sure you stay balanced and feel your hips and hamstrings loosen up.

5. Lower the Leg: Carefully lower your leg back to where it started.

6. Do the same thing with your left leg.

7. Switch the legs: Repeat this process several times, switching which leg you lift each time.

Tips and Changes:

- Maintain Alignment: Stand up straight and keep your upper body still. When you lift your leg, don't lean forward.

- Controlled Movement: Make sure that you have full control over how high and low you lift your leg.

- Focus on Breathing: Time your breath with the movement by breathing in as you lift your leg and breathing out as you lower it.

- Change Height: Lift your leg up as high as you can without stretching. The goal is on moving with control and using your muscles.

- Boost the Challenge: As your strength grows, you can hold your leg up for longer periods of time or add ankle weights for extra challenge.

CHAIR SHUFFLE LEG

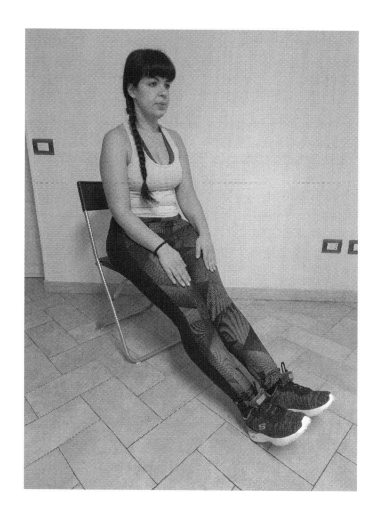

Instructions

1. Sit in a chair, feet flat on the floor, a bit apart from each other.

2. Lean back slightly in your chair and hold the sides for balance.

3. Lift your feet just a bit off the ground.

4. Start moving your legs in and out, like shuffling. One foot goes out while the other comes in.

5. Do this for a few seconds or as long as comfortable, then rest.

Tips and Changes:

- Start slow and increase the pace as you feel more comfortable.

- Keep your back straight while doing the exercise.

- Breathe normally, don't hold your breath.

- If you feel tired, stop and rest before continuing.

- If lifting both feet is hard, try lifting one foot at a time.

STEP OUT

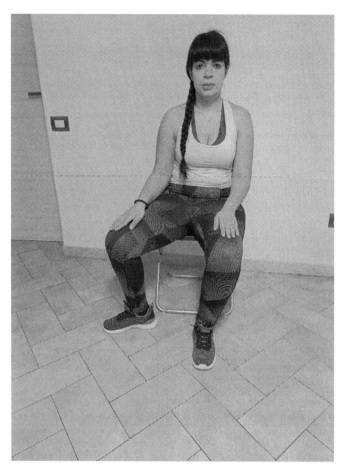 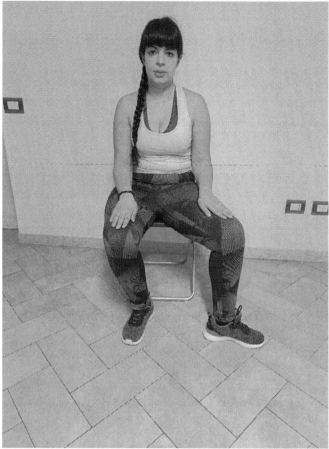

Instructions

1. Sit in a chair with your feet flat on the floor and close together.

2. Hold onto the sides of the chair for balance.

3. Step your right foot out to the side, keeping your left foot in place.

4. Bring your right foot back to the starting position.

5. Repeat with your left foot, stepping out to the side.

6. Continue alternating between your right and left foot.

Tips and Changes:

- Move at a comfortable pace and don't rush.

- Keep your back straight and avoid leaning to the sides.

- If it's hard to step far out, start with small steps and gradually increase.

- Breathe evenly throughout the exercise.

- For more challenge, increase the speed or step further out.

CURLS

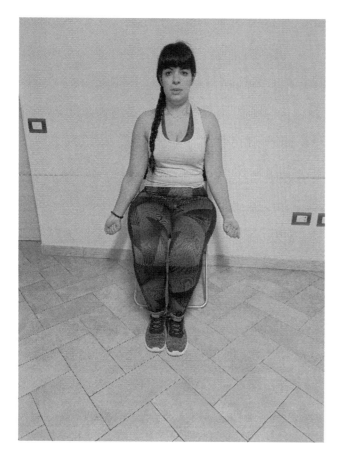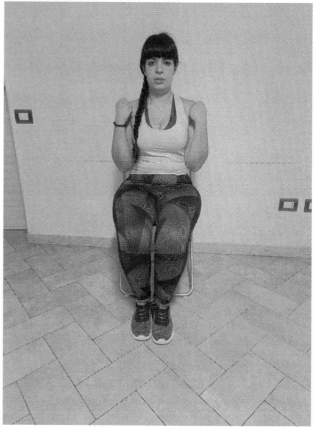

Instructions

1. Sit in a chair with your feet flat on the floor, hip-width apart.

2. Hold a small weight or a water bottle in each hand, arms at your sides, palms facing forward.

3. Bend your elbows and lift the weights towards your shoulders.

4. Lower your arms back to the starting position.

5. Repeat the motion for several repetitions.

Tips and Changes:

- Move your arms slowly and with control.

- Keep your back straight and avoid leaning back as you lift the weights.

- If you don't have weights, you can use household items like water bottles or cans.

- Breathe out as you lift the weights and breathe in as you lower them.

- If it's too hard with weights, try doing the curls without any weight. To make it harder, use heavier weights or increase the number of repetitions.

SEATED TOE TAPS

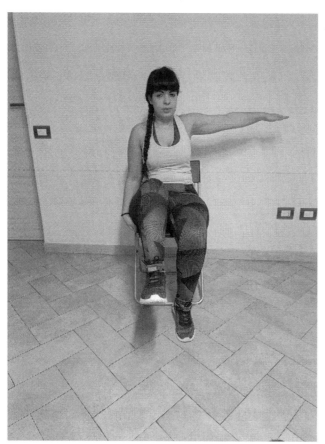 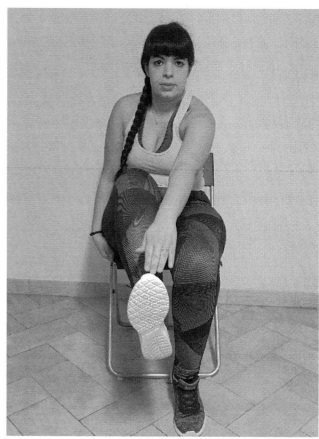

Instructions

1. Sit in a chair with your feet flat on the floor and knees bent.

2. Keep your back straight and hold onto the sides of the chair for balance.

3. Lift your right foot and tap the floor with your toes.

4. Place your right foot back on the floor.

5. Repeat the motion with your left foot.

6. Alternate between your right and left foot for several repetitions.

Tips and Changes:

- Keep the movements light and quick, like you're tapping to music.
- Stay upright in your chair, avoiding leaning back or forward.
- If lifting your foot is difficult, try sliding your foot forward instead of lifting.
- Breathe normally and try to establish a rhythmic pattern with your taps.
- To make it easier, slow down the pace. For more of a challenge, increase the speed or add ankle weights.

SEATED KNEE TO NOSE

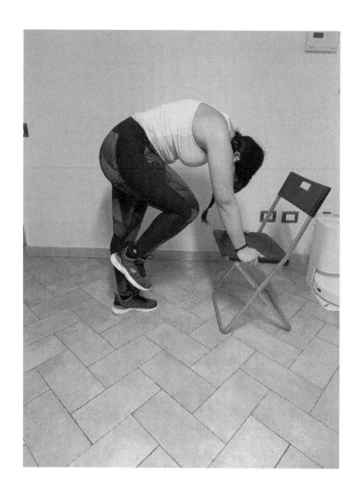 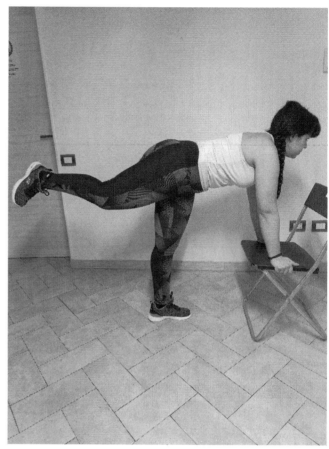

Instructions

1. Stand with your feet in front of the chair.

2. Place your hands on the chair for support.

3. Inhale and bend your right leg, bringing the knee up between your hands.

4. Exhale and stretch the leg out behind you.

5. Repeat this movement about 4 times, moving slowly with each exhalation. You can exhale through your mouth.

6. After completing with the right leg, switch and repeat the sequence with the left leg.

Tips and Changes:

- When extending your leg behind you, be careful not to overstretch.

- To connect with your abdominal muscles, consider placing one hand on your belly as you move through the sequence.

- Focus on smooth and controlled movements, coordinating each movement with your breath.

LEG PUSH-UP

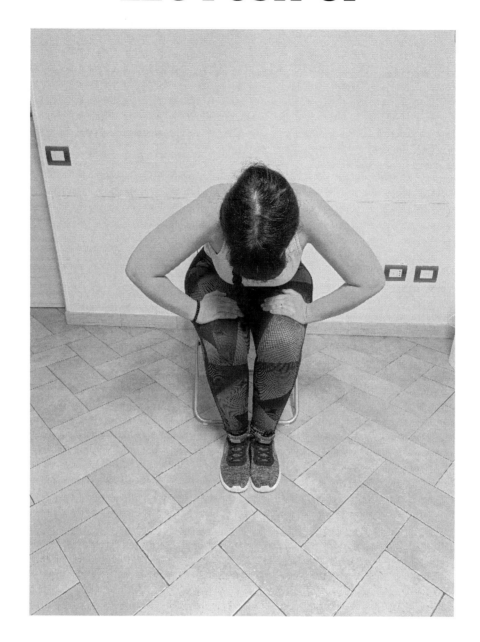

Instructions

1. Sit on a chair with your feet on the floor, a bit apart.

2. Hold the sides of the chair.

3. Lift one leg straight in front of you, up to knee height.

4. Push your leg up a little, like you're pressing something.

5. Hold it there for a bit, then lower it down.

6. Do the same with your other leg.

7. Keep switching legs and do it several times.

Tips and Changes:

- Move slowly and don't rush.

- If lifting high is hard, lift your leg just a little.

- To make it harder, hold your leg up longer or use ankle weights.

- Sit straight and don't lean back while lifting your leg.

STAND HAMSTRING CURL

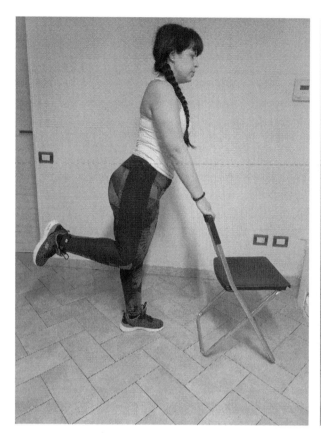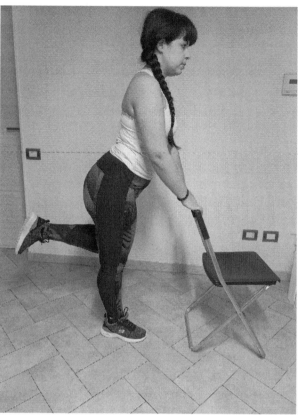

Instructions

1. Stand up straight near a chair for support.

2. Hold onto the back of the chair.

3. Lift your right foot off the floor, bending your knee.

4. Bring your heel towards your seat, like you're curling your leg back.

5. Hold for a moment, then lower your foot back down.

6. Do the same with your left leg.

7. Keep switching legs and repeat several times.

Tips and Changes:

- Do this slowly and don't rush.

- If it's hard to curl your leg all the way back, just go as far as you can.

- For more of a challenge, don't hold onto the chair.

- Stand tall and don't lean on the chair too much.

SEATED KICK AND PUNCH

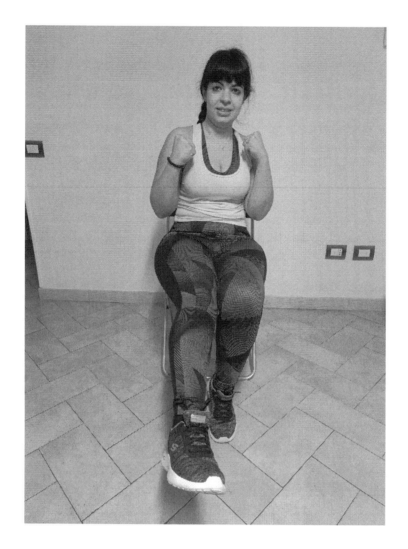

Instructions

1. Sit on a chair with your feet flat on the ground and hands by your sides.

2. Lift your right leg and kick forward, at the same time punch forward with your left hand.

3. Bring your leg and arm back to the starting position.

4. Now lift your left leg and kick, and punch with your right hand.

5. Keep alternating kicks and punches between legs and opposite arms.

6. Do this for several repetitions.

Tips and Changes:

- Keep your movements controlled.

- If kicking high is hard, start with lower kicks.

- Breathe out when you kick and punch, breathe in when you return to starting position.

- For more challenge, speed up your kicks and punches.

- Sit up straight and try not to lean back in the chair.

SEATED MARCH

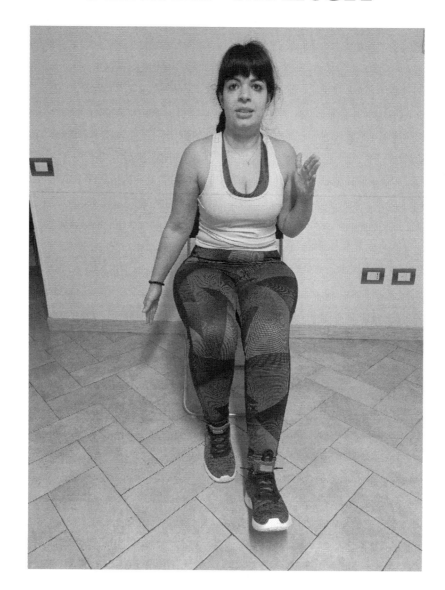

Instructions

1. Sit in a chair, feet on the floor, and back straight.

2. Lift your right knee up, like you're marching.

3. Put it down and then lift your left knee.

4. Keep lifting your knees, like marching on the spot.

5. Do this for some time, like a few minutes.

Tips and Changes:

- Move at your own pace, not too fast.

- If lifting your knee high is hard, lift it just a little.

- For more challenge, lift your knees higher or march faster.

- Keep your back straight and don't lean back.

TORSO TWIST

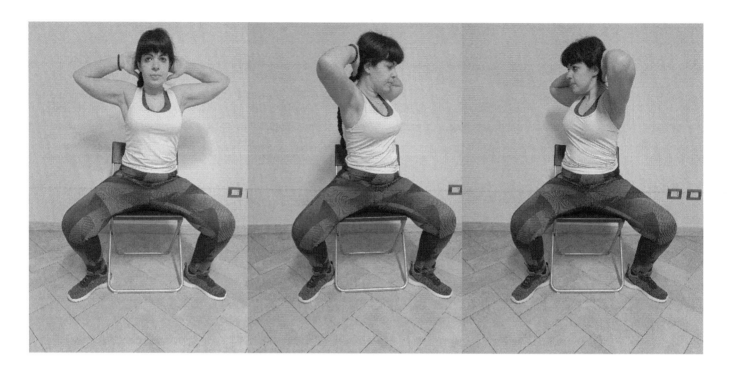

Instructions

1. Sit in a chair with feet flat on the floor and back straight.

2. Place your right hand on your left knee and your left hand behind you for support.

3. Twist your upper body to the left, starting from your waist.

4. Hold for a few seconds, then return to facing forward.

5. Repeat on the other side, placing your left hand on your right knee and twisting to the right.

Tips and Changes:

- Twist gently, don't force it.

- Keep your back straight while twisting.

- If it's hard to twist far, do a smaller twist.

- Breathe out as you twist, breathe in as you come back.

- For a bigger challenge, twist without using your hands for

   support.

L AND KICK

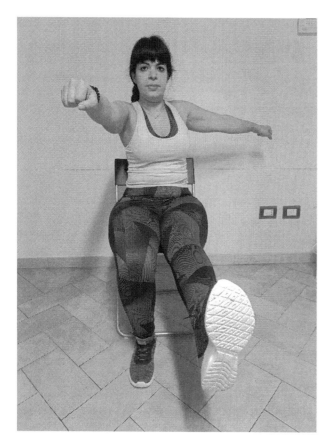 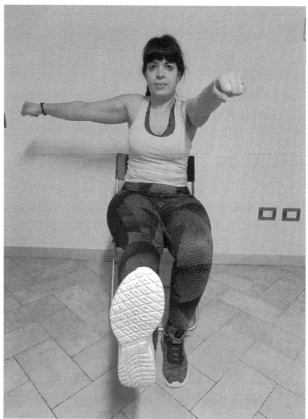

Instructions

1. Sit in a chair, back straight and feet flat on the floor.

2. Lift your right knee up to hip height, making an "L" shape with your leg.

3. Then, extend your right leg out straight, like you're kicking.

4. Bend your knee back to the "L" shape.

5. Lower your leg down to starting position.

6. Repeat with your left leg.

7. Alternate between your right and left leg for several repetitions.

Tips and Changes:

- Move slowly and with control.

- If fully extending your leg is hard, just stretch it a bit.

- For more challenge, hold your leg out for a few seconds before bending.

- Keep sitting up straight and don't lean back in the chair.

CROSS PUNCHES

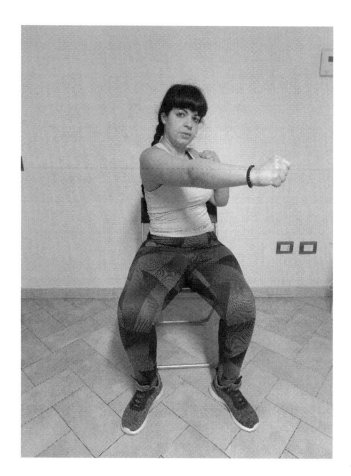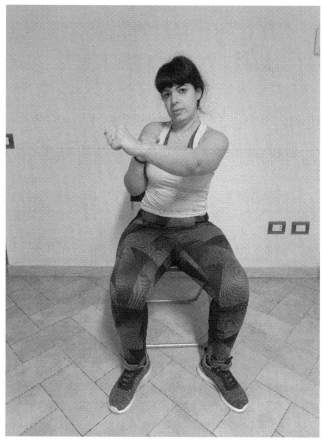

Instructions

1. Sit in a chair with your feet flat on the ground and back straight.

2. Clench your fists and hold them up near your face.

3. Twist your torso to the right and punch your left fist across your body.

4. Bring your fist back, then twist and punch your right fist across your body to the left.

5. Keep alternating punches to the right and left.

Tips and Changes:

- Punch with control, not too fast.

- Twist your body with each punch.

- If twisting is hard, just punch straight forward.

- Breathe out when you punch, breathe in when you come back.

- For more challenge, punch faster or add small weights in your hands.

STARS

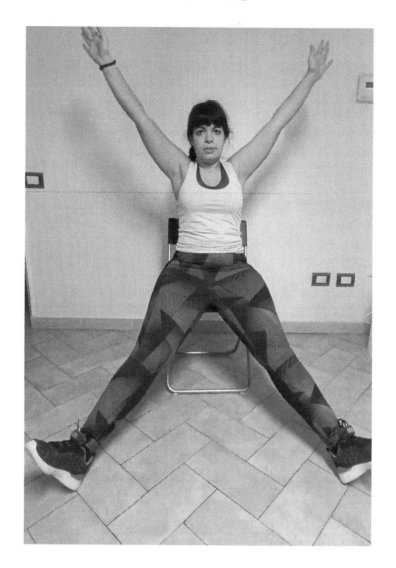

Instructions

1. Sit in a chair with your feet on the floor and your back straight.
2. Lift your right arm and left leg at the same time, reaching out to the side.

3. Bring them back down and then lift your left arm and right leg, reaching out.

4. Keep alternating, like you're creating a star shape with each lift.

5. Do this movement for several repetitions.

Tips and Changes:

- Move in a steady and controlled way.

- If lifting your arm and leg high is tough, just lift them a little bit.

- Breathe in as you lift your arm and leg, breathe out as you lower them.

- To make it easier, you can just lift an arm or a leg at one time.

- For more challenge, lift your arm and leg higher or do it faster.

UPPERCUTS

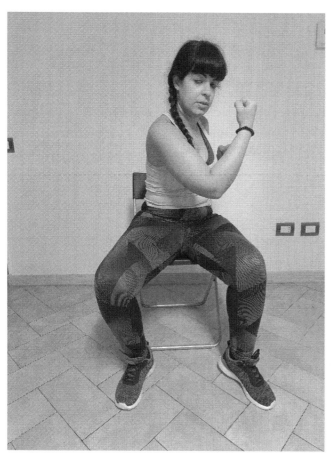 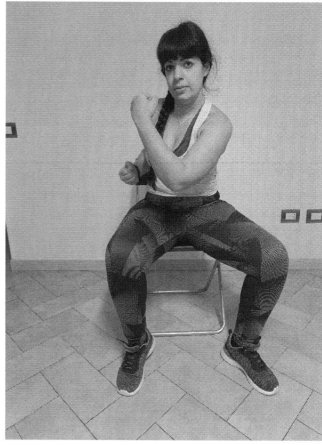

Instructions

1. Sit in a chair with your feet flat on the floor and back straight.

2. Clench your fists and hold them near your chin.

3. Bend your elbow to lift your right fist up in a swift, upward motion, as if you're aiming under an imaginary chin.

4. Bring your right fist back to starting position.

5. Do the same with your left fist, lifting it in an uppercut motion.

6. Alternate between your right and left fists, performing the uppercut motion.

Tips and Changes:

- Do the uppercuts with control; don't do them too fast.
- Keep your wrists straight to avoid injury.
- If full uppercuts are hard, do smaller, gentler motions.
- Breathe out as you do the uppercut, breathe in as you return to starting position.
- For more challenge, speed up your uppercuts or use small hand weights.

BUTTERFLY

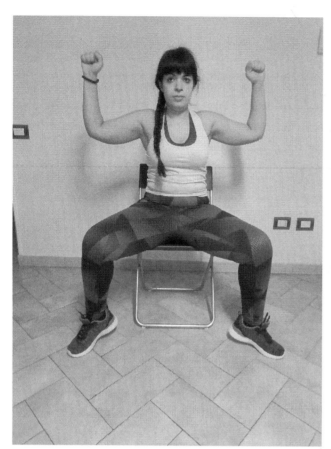 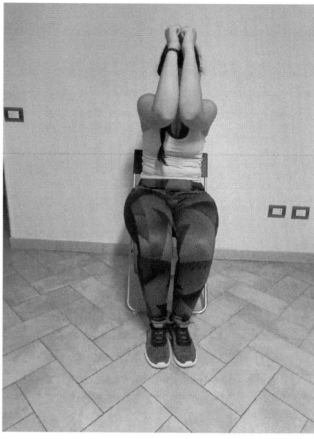

Instructions

1. Sit in a chair with your feet flat on the ground and back straight.

2. Bring the soles of your feet together in front of you, letting your knees drop to the sides.

3. Hold your feet with your hands and sit up tall.

4. Gently bounce your knees up and down, like the wings of a butterfly.

5. Do this for a few seconds or as long as comfortable.

Tips and Changes:

- Move your knees gently, don't force them down.
- Keep your back straight and avoid leaning forward.
- If it's hard to bring your feet together, keep them a bit apart.
- Breathe normally as you move your knees.
- To make it easier, don't bounce your knees, just hold the position. For more stretch, gently press down on your thighs.

STEP OUT AND PRESS

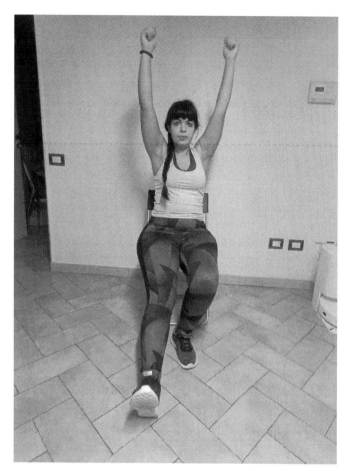 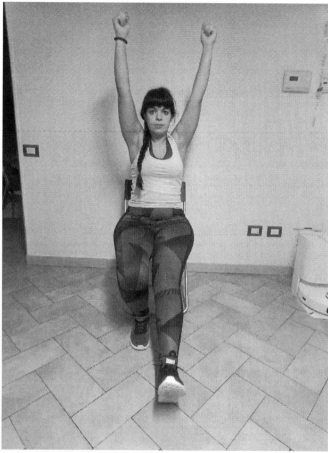

Instructions

1. Sit in a chair with your feet flat on the ground and back straight.

2. Hold a small weight or water bottle in each hand, near your shoulders.

3. Step your right foot out to the side.

4. As you step out, press the weights up above your head.

5. Bring your right foot back and lower the weights to your shoulders.

6. Repeat the same on the left side.

7. Alternate stepping out with each leg and pressing the weights.

Tips and Changes:

- Move smoothly and with control.

- Keep your back straight as you step out and press.

- If using weights is hard, do it without them.

- Breathe out as you press up, breathe in as you come back.

- For more challenge, use heavier weights or increase the pace.

TRAINING PLANS

In this chapter, we're going to talk about training plans. These are like your road maps for chair yoga and gentle exercises. If you're new to this or have been doing it for a while, these plans will help you get the most out of your workouts.

What Are Training Plans?

Think of training plans as special guides for your exercises. They're not just random exercises thrown together. Instead, they're carefully picked to help you get stronger, more flexible, and feel better, step by step. And the best part? Chair yoga is for everyone. So, no matter how old you are or how fit you feel, there's a plan just for you.Make It Your Own:

You can fit these plans into your day, no matter how busy you are. Remember, doing a little bit every day can make a big difference.

Let's Get Going:

So, are you ready to start? These training plans are not just about getting fit; they're about feeling great and having fun. Let's explore these plans together and find the joy in moving and stretching!

SUNRISE SEQUENCE

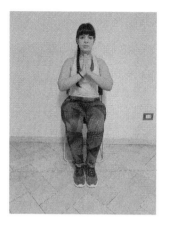

FREE TIME

PRAYER POSE

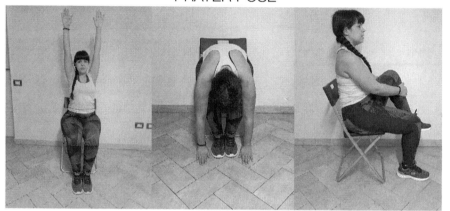

10 REPS

HANDS UP   FOLD POSE   LOW LUNGE

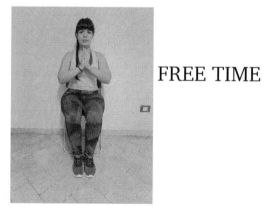

FREE TIME

PRAYER POSE

SOFT START STRETCH

SIDE STRETCH LEFT   SIDE STRETCH RIGHT   SIDE TWIST

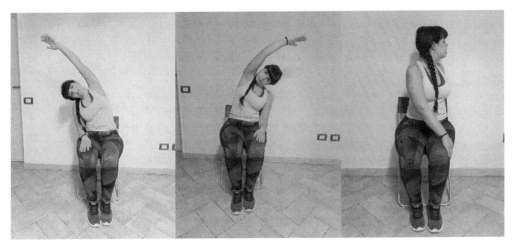

5 reps   5 reps   3 reps

CAT COW   SHOULDER CIRCLES   CACTUS ARMS

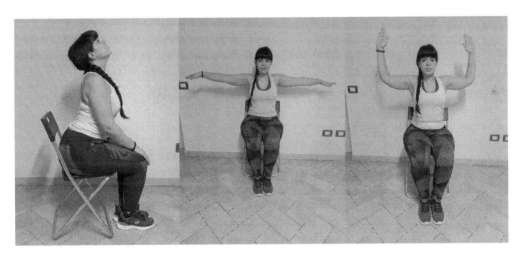

5 REPS   30 SEC   8 REPS

SOOTHING BACK EASE

CAT COW	COBRA POSE	SIDE TWIST LEFT AND RIGHT

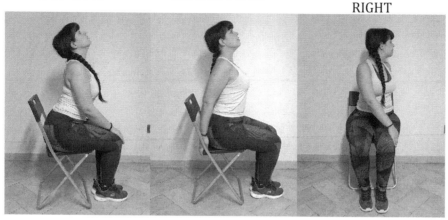

5 REPS	3 REPS	3 REPS

SAGE TWIST RIGHT	SAGE TWIST LEFT	COBRA POSE

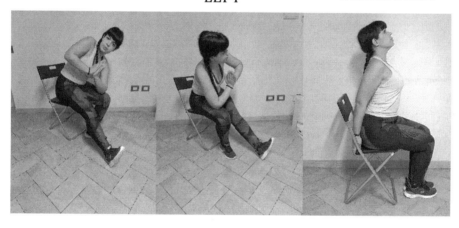

HOLD 20 SEC	HOLD 20 SEC	3 REPS

HANDS UP	FOLD POSE

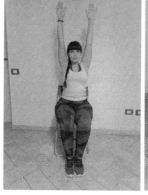 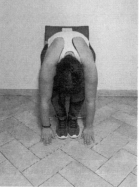

5 REPS

CALM NECK AND SHOULDERS

SUN BREATHS

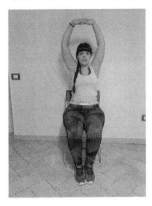

3 REPS

| NECK ROLLS | UP AND DOWN | SHOULDER CIRCLES |

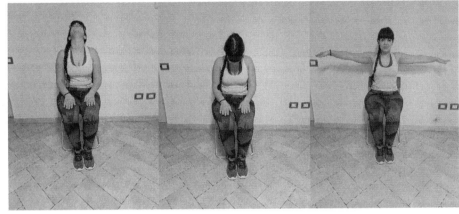

| 40 SEC | 5 REPS | 30 SEC |

| HANDS UP | FOLD POSE |

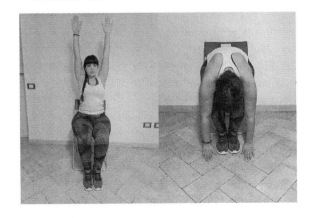

| 5 REPS | 5 REPS |

LEGS RELIEF

LOW LUNGE LEFT

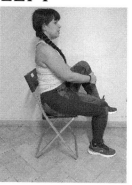

30 SEC

LOW LUNGE RIGHT

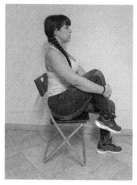

30 SEC

ONE LEGGED RIGHT

15 SEC

ONE LEGGED LEFT

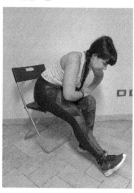

15 SEC

PIGEON STRETCH RIGHT

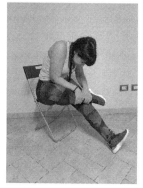

15 SEC

PIGEON STRETCH LEFT

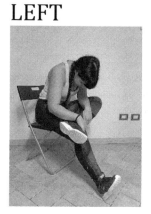

15 SEC

FOOT FLEXING RIGHT

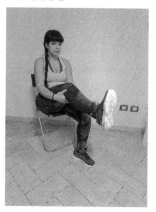

8 REPS

FOOT FLEXING LEFT

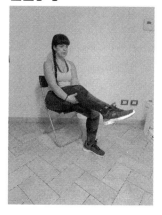

8 REPS

MUSCLE TONING 1

PRAYER POSE

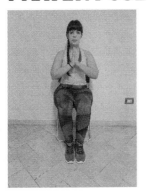

FREE TIME

SUN BREATH

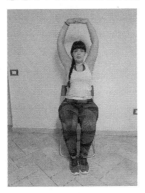

5 REPS

ASSISTED LEG EXTENSION RIGHT

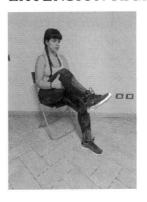

8 REPS

SAGE TWIST LEFT

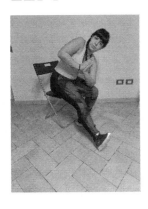

15 SEC

SAGE TWIST RIGHT

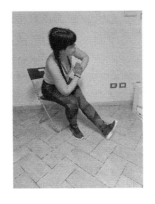

15 SEC

ASSISTED LEG EXTENSION LEFT

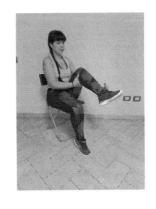

8 REPS

BOAT

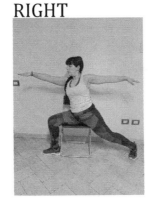

10 SEC X 3 REPS

WARRIOR POSE RIGHT

15 SEC

WARRIOR POSE LEFT

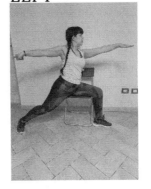

15 SEC

MUSCLE TONING 2

PRAYER POSE

HUMBLE WARRIOR POSE LEFT

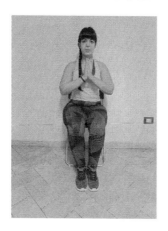
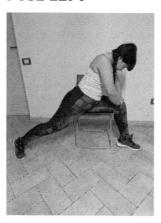

FREE TIME

15 SEC

ASSISTED LEG EXTENSION RIGHT

WARRIOR POSE LEFT

WARRIOR POSE RIGHT

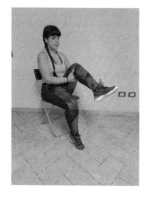
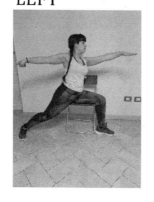
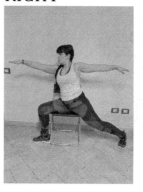

8 REPS

15 SEC

15 SEC

HIGH LUNGE LEFT

HIGH LUNGE RIGHT

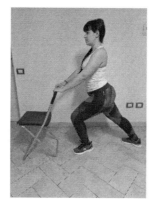
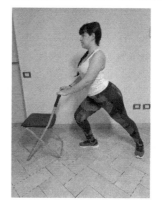

20 SEC

20 SEC

LEGS SCULPTING 1

SEATED MARCH

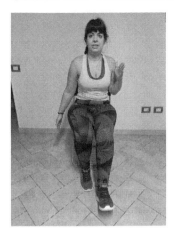

30 SEC

LEG RAISES
LEFT

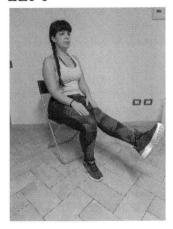

8 REPS

LEG RAISES
RIGHT

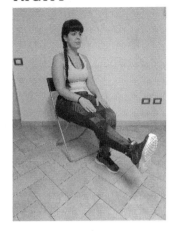

8 REPS

CALF RAISES

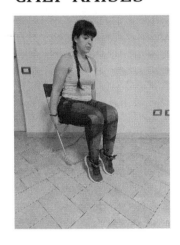

10 REPS

ALTERNATIVE
CALF RAISES LEFT

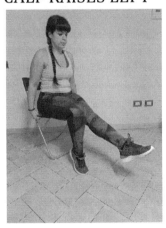

8 REPS

ALTERNATIVE CALF
RAISES RIGHT

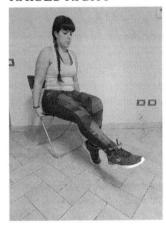

8 REPS

STEP OUT RIGHT

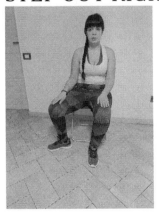

8 REPS

STEP OUT LEFT

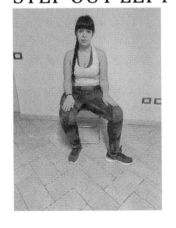

8 REPS

SEATED MARCH

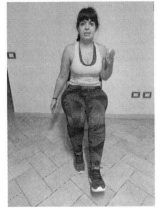

30 SEC

121

LEGS SCULPTING 2

SEATED MARCH

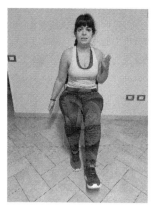

30 SEC

STEP OUT RIGHT

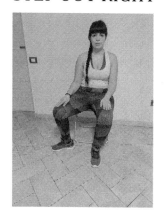

8 REPS

STEP OUT RIGHT

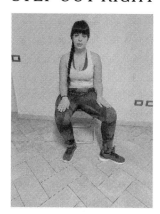

8 REPS

SEATED TOE TAPS ALTERNATE

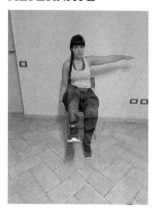

6 REPS X LEG

CHAIR SQUATS

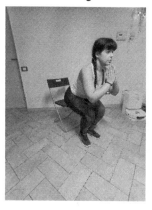

5 REPS

STANDING HAMSTRING RIGHT

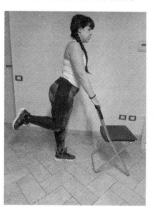

15 REPS

STANDING HAMSTRING LEFT

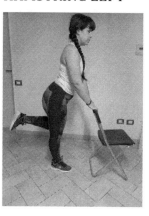

15 REPS

SEATED MARCH

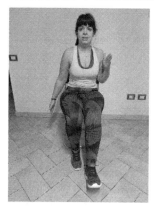

30 SEC

LEGS SCULPTING 3

SEATED MARCH

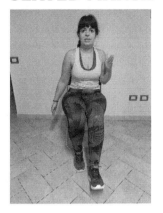

30 SEC

CHAIR SHUFFLE

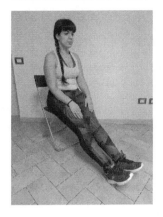

8 REPS

LEG RAISES LEFT

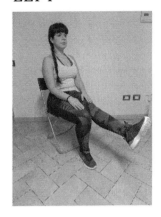

8 REPS

LEG RAISES RIGHT

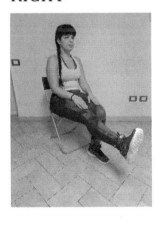

8 REPS

CHAIR SQUATS

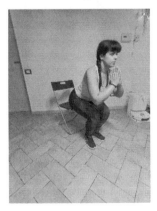

5 REPS

MOUNTAIN POSE OLB RIGHT

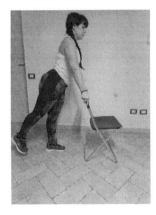

15 REPS

MOUNTAIN POSE OLB LEFT

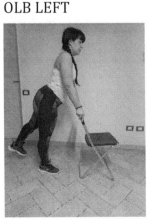

15 REPS

SEATED MARCH

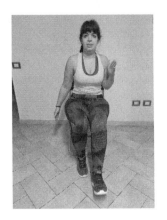

30 SEC

TOTAL BODY SCULPTING 1

LEG RAISES LEFT

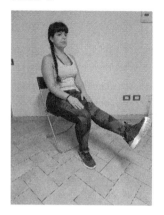

8 REPS

LEG RAISES RIGHT

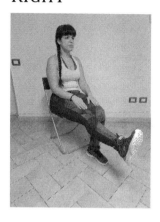

8 REPS

CALF RAISES ALTERNATE

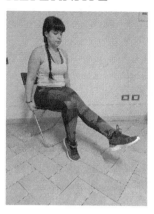

8 REPS

CHAIR SQUATS

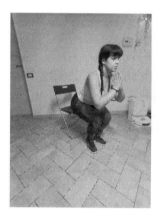

5 REPS

KNEE TO NOSE RIGHT

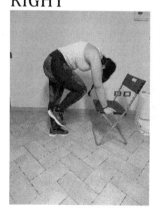

8 REPS

KNEE TO NOSE LEFT

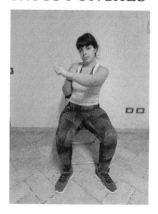

8 REPS

BUTTERFLY

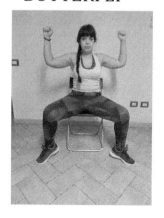

30 SEC

CROSS PUNCHES

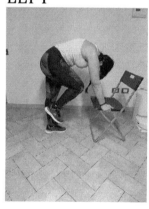

40 SEC

TOTAL BODY SCULPTING 2

MOUNTAIN POSE
OLB RIGHT

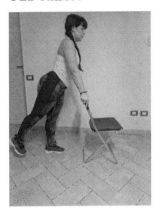

MOUNTAIN POSE
OLB LEFT

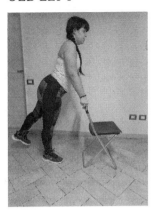

15 REPS

15 REPS

STANDING
HAMSTRING RIGHT

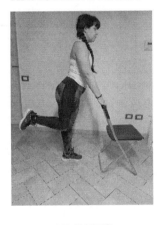

STANDING
HAMSTRING LEFT

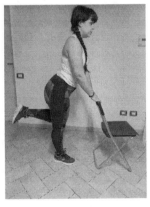

CALF RAISES
ALTERNATE

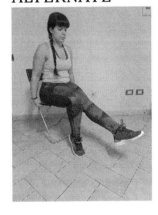

15 REPS

15 REPS

8 REPS

STEP OUT RIGHT

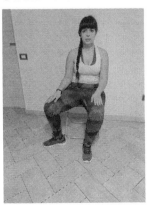

UPEERCUTS

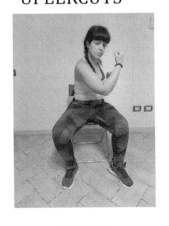

STEP OUT AND
PRESS

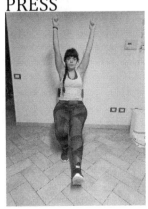

8 REPS

30 SEC

30 SEC

TOTAL BODY SCULPTING 3

KNEE TO NOSE LEFT

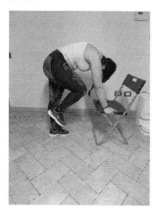

8 REPS

KNEE TO NOSE RIGHT

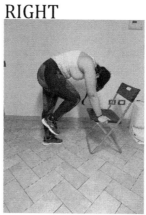

8 REPS

MOUNTAIN POSE OLB RIGHT

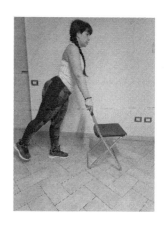

15 REPS

MOUNTAIN POSE OLB LEFT

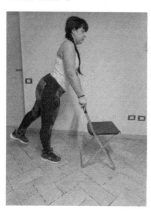

15 REPS

CHAIR SHUFFLE

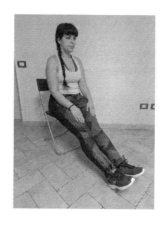

8 REPS

CACTUS ARMS

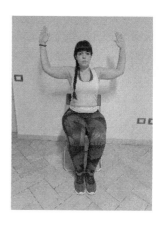

8 REPS

CROSS PUNCHES

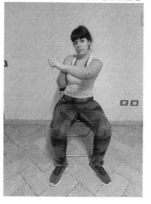

40 SEC

UPEERCUTS

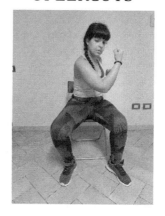

30 SEC

CARDIO 1

SEATED KICK AND PUNCH

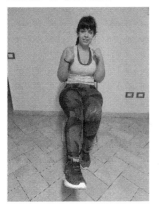

30 SEC

TORSO TWIST

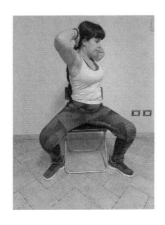

30 SEC

REST

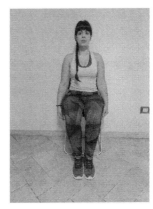

30 SEC

SEATED MARCH

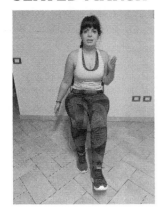

30 SEC

STARS

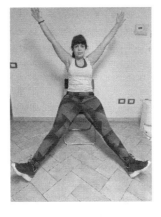

30 SEC

REST

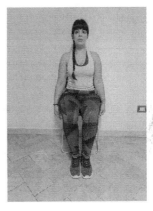

30 SEC

L AND KICK

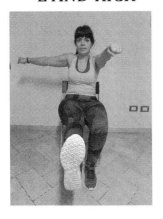

30 SEC

SEATED MARCH

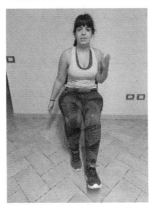

30 SEC

CARDIO 2

SEATED MARCH

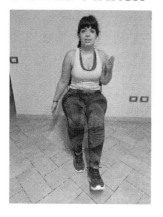

30 SEC

UPEERCUTS

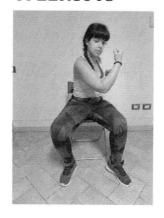

30 SEC

REST

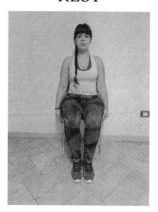

30 SEC

SEATED MARCH

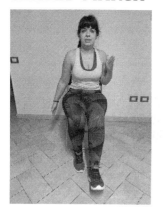

30 SEC

CROSS PUNCHES

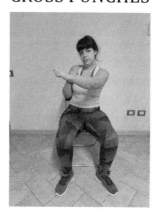

40 SEC

REST

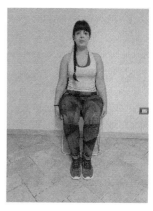

30 SEC

SEATED MARCH

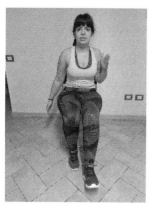

30 SEC

SEATED KICK AND PUNCH

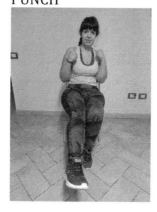

30 SEC

CARDIO 3

L AND KICK

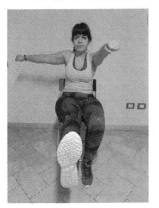

30 SEC

STARS

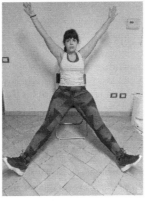

30 SEC

REST

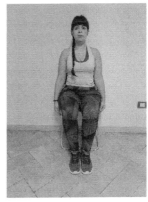

30 SEC

SEATED MARCH

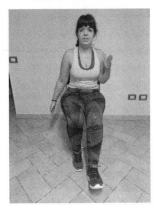

30 SEC

SEATED KICK AND PUNCH

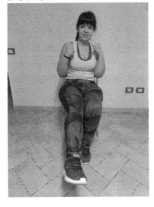

30 SEC

REST

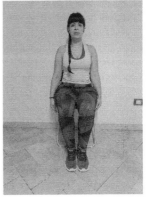

30 SEC

BUTTERFLY

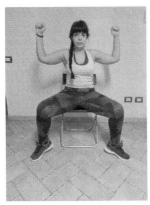

30 SEC

STEP OUT AND PRESS

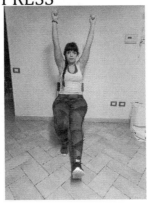

30 SEC

CARDIO 4

SEATED MARCH

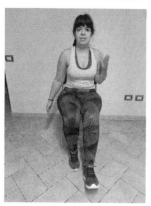

30 SEC

UPEERCUTS

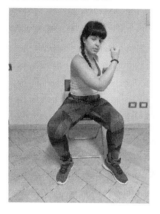

30 SEC

CROSS PUNCHES

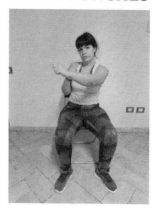

40 SEC

SEATED MARCH

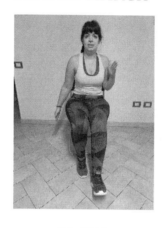

30 SEC

REST

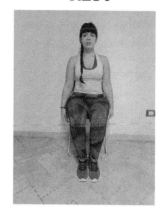

30 SEC

REST

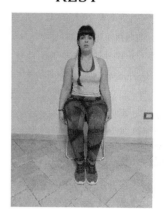

30 SEC

SEATED KICK AND
PUNCH

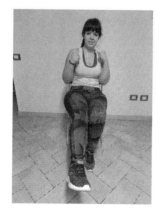

30 SEC

SEATED MARCH

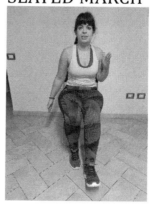

30 SEC

CARDIO 5

STARS

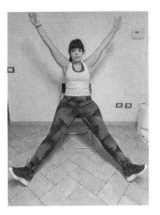

30 SEC

STEP OUT AND PRESS

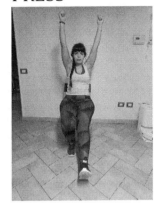

30 SEC

REST

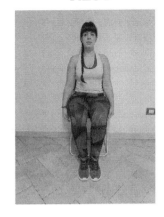

30 SEC

TORSO TWIST

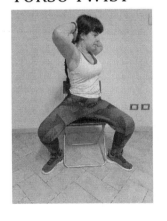

30 SEC

SEATED KICK AND PUNCH

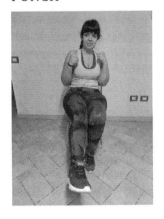

30 SEC

REST

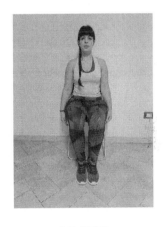

30 SEC

L AND KICK

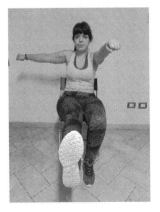

30 SEC

BUTTERFLY

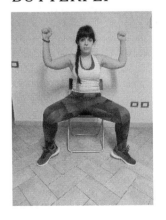

30 SEC

28 DAY CHALLENGE

28-Day Challenge: Your Path to Transformation

Welcome to the "28-Day Challenge," an exciting journey designed to transform your fitness and well-being! This challenge is a carefully structured program that combines various workouts to enhance your strength, flexibility, and cardiovascular health. Here's how to approach it:

Getting Started:

- Commitment: Dedicate yourself to the next 28 days. Consistency is key to seeing results.

- Schedule: Plan a specific time each day for your workout. Consistency helps turn exercise into a habit.

The Workouts:

- Each day features a different focus, from gentle warm-ups and stretching to more dynamic exercises like cardio and full-body toning.

- The routines gradually increase in intensity, so you'll build strength and stamina as you progress through the challenge.

Tips for Success:

- Listen to Your Body: While it's good to push yourself, don't ignore your body's signals. Rest if you need to.

- Stay Hydrated and Eat Healthily: Nutrition and hydration are crucial for recovery and energy.

- Track Your Progress: Keep a journal or use an app to track your workouts and how you feel. This can be very motivating.

Support:

- You're not alone! Join our online community for support, tips, and sharing your progress.

- Celebrate small victories. Every day you complete is a step closer to your goal.

Conclusion:

At the end of the 28 days, not only will you notice improvements in your physical fitness, but you'll also likely see changes in your mental well-being. Approach each day as an opportunity to grow stronger and more confident. Let's get started!

Week 1

- Day 1: Warm-Up: Soft Start Stretch; Workout: Total Body Sculpting 1

- Day 2: Warm-Up: Soothing Back Ease; Workout: Legs Sculpting 1

- Day 3: Warm-Up: Legs Relief; Workout: Cardio 1

- Day 4: Warm-Up: Calm Neck and Shoulders; Workout: Total Body Sculpting 2

- Day 5: Rest Day

- Day 6: Warm-Up: Soft Start Stretch; Workout: Legs Sculpting 2

- Day 7: Warm-Up: Soothing Back Ease; Workout: Cardio 2

Week 2

- Day 8: Warm-Up: Legs Relief; Workout: Total Body Sculpting 3

- Day 9: Warm-Up: Calm Neck and Shoulders; Workout: Legs Sculpting 3

- Day 10: Rest Day

- Day 11: Warm-Up: Soft Start Stretch; Workout: Cardio 3

- Day 12: Warm-Up: Soothing Back Ease; Workout: Total Body Sculpting 1

- Day 13: Warm-Up: Legs Relief; Workout: Cardio 4

- Day 14: Rest Day

Week 3

- Day 15: Warm-Up: Calm Neck and Shoulders; Workout: Total Body Sculpting 2

- Day 16: Warm-Up: Soft Start Stretch; Workout: Legs Sculpting 1

- Day 17: Warm-Up: Soothing Back Ease; Workout: Cardio 5

- Day 18: Rest Day

- Day 19: Warm-Up: Legs Relief; Workout: Total Body Sculpting 3

- Day 20: Warm-Up: Calm Neck and Shoulders; Workout: Legs Sculpting 2

- Day 21: Rest Day

Week 4

- Day 22: Warm-Up: Soft Start Stretch; Workout: Cardio 1

- Day 23: Warm-Up: Soothing Back Ease; Workout: Total Body Sculpting 1

- Day 24: Warm-Up: Legs Relief; Workout: Legs Sculpting 3

- Day 25: Rest Day

- Day 26: Warm-Up: Calm Neck and Shoulders; Workout: Cardio 2

- Day 27: Warm-Up: Soft Start Stretch; Workout: Total Body Sculpting 2

- Day 28: Rest Day and Reflection

VIDEOS!

Thank you for choosing to purchase this book!

This is a QR code that gives you access to a series of video tutorials.
These videos cover each exercise described in the book, providing you
with visual guidance and additional tips to ensure you get the most out of
your workouts. Simply scan the QR code with your smartphone or tablet,
and you'll be directed to our specially curated collection of video tutorials.
We hope these resources will help you deepen your understanding of the
exercises and enrich your overall fitness journey.

Thank you once again for your trust and commitment to your health and
well-being. Let's get moving!

Scan this QR code!

EXTRA BONUS

Unlock Your Exclusive Bonus: Wall Pilates Workouts - Yours FREE!

Dear Valued Customer,

Your journey with our product has, we hope, begun to transform your daily routine for the better. As you continue to explore and enjoy its benefits, we have an exciting opportunity for you to deepen your wellness journey even further.

If you liked our book let us know with an Amazon review & receive a complimentary book on Wall Pilates!

As a token of our gratitude for your time and insights, we're offering you an exclusive bonus:

• A Digital Copy of "**Wall Pilates Workouts**" - This comprehensive guide is designed to complement your current practice, introducing you to the transformative world of wall pilates. Whether you're a beginner or looking to enhance your routine, this book promises to unlock new dimensions of strength, flexibility, and wellness.

Scan this QR code to download your awesome book!

Don't miss out on this exclusive offer to elevate your practice and discover the power of wall pilates.

Made in the USA
Columbia, SC
02 June 2024

36541043R00076